Handbook of Statistical Methods

Single Subject Design

Handbook of Statistical Methods

Single Subject Design

Eike Satake, Ph.D.
Vinoth Jagaroo, Ph.D
David L. Maxwell, Ph.D

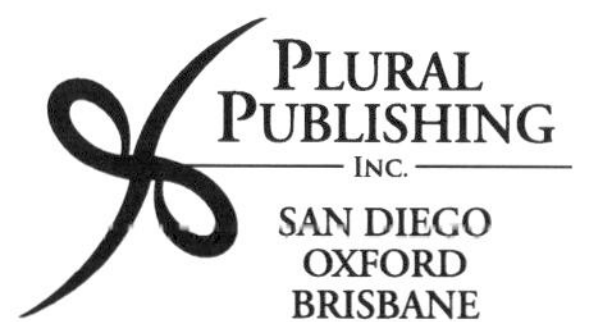

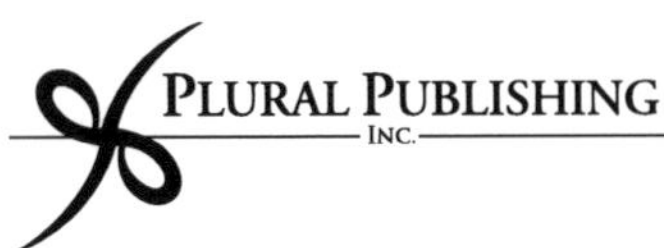

5521 Ruffin Road
San Diego, CA 92123

e-mail: info@pluralpublishing.com
Web site: http://www.pluralpublishing.com

Library of Congress Cataloging-in-Publication Data:

Satake, Eike.
 Handbook of statistical methods : single subject design / Eike Satake, Vinoth Jagaroo and David L. Maxwell.
     p. ; cm.
 Includes bibliographical references and index.
 ISBN-13: 978-1-59756-098-6 (alk. paper)
 ISBN-10: 1-59756-098-7 (alk. paper)
  1. Clinical medicine—Statistical methods—Handbooks, manuals, etc. 2. Single subject research—Handbooks, manuals, etc.
  [DNLM: 1. Statistics as Topic—methods. 2. Research Design. 3. Sample Size. WA 950 S253h 2007] I. Jagaroo, Vinoth. II. Maxwell, David L. III. Title.
 R853.S7.S333 2007
  610.72'7—dc22
                                                                              2007051119

Contents

Preface

In the behavioral, health, and clinical sciences, single subject designs have increasingly become important tools for determining the efficacy of a treatment. Studies utilizing single subject designs can be found across a variety of clinical areas. Treatment interventions in stroke, speech-language disorders, hearing loss, autism, attention deficit and hyperactivity disorder, counseling and rehabilitation psychology, various avenues of occupational therapy; performance interventions in sports psychology; nursing interventions; and pharmacologic trials and interventions are among the many clinical contexts where single subject designs are employed.

In recent years, there have been even greater calls for the use of single subject designs. Interest in single subject designs is generally driven by a number of factors, ranging from limited numbers of subjects to certain inherent advantages of single subject designs: In the behavioral and clinical sciences, it is often the case that availability of large numbers of subjects for the study of certain problems can be limited. When a large number of subjects, often required to fulfill the criteria of group designs, is not available, single subject designs provide alternative methods of statistical validation. A second advantage of single subject designs over group designs is that the methods employed are more adaptable to many clinical research problems in which the main interest is in assessing the effect of treatment on individual patients over an extended period of time. Such specificity of focus allows for predicting whether or not an individual participant may or may not benefit from a particular intervention. In other words, the design has more capability for examination of intersubject variability over group design experiment. In group design, the variability is statistically derived and often some participants may not show any improvement despite the fact that the results show statistically significant improvement overall. Third, single subject designs are well adapted for satisfying the goals of quality assurance established by public and private health care providers. Questions pertaining to both the short-term and long-term benefits of various treatment interventions can be answered because of the ability of such designs to profile treatment results for individual clients. Last, statistically speaking, single subject design allows us to more accurately identify a covariate (confounding variable) than group designs. Therefore, we can perform the analysis of covariance (ANCOVA) to control the influence of extraneous variables and experimenter bias much more easily than with group designs.

Even as the use of single subjects designs (SSDs) becomes more widespread, the vast majority of typical research and statistical methods textbooks still fall short in providing sufficient direction and information about single subject designs. One of the main reasons for this is that the methods of data analysis in single subject designs are still foreign to most investigators, clinical practitioners, and students. Single subject designs are often described in a manner and that does not provide adequate detail on methods of analysis. This is somewhat incongruous with the ever growing popularity of SSDs. We have therefore developed this practical guide—a book that describes the most commonly used approaches in analyzing and interpreting single subject data.

This handbook is aimed largely at graduate students preparing for professional work in clinical/health sciences and practitioners who wish to enhance their knowledge of clinical research. It can serve as a supplement to a traditional course textbook and/or a formal lecture series given to graduate students and clinical practitioners who have some knowledge about single subject research. It can play a role in a seminar series for researchers, students, and clinical practitioners, freeing them from the heavier didactic aspects of the teaching/learning environment and thereby enabling more discussion of SSDs. It may also be used as a vehicle for a refresher course or an independent study program for those who wish to revisit the subject matter.

As a handbook, this guide describes the essential theory and methods of SSDs with emphasis on data analysis. It also describes some clinical scenarios through which the application of these designs is practically illustrated. The book is divided into two sections.

Part I presents the historical and theoretical foundations of SSDs. It uses a straightforward question-and-answer format to:

1. Introduce each of the single subject designs.
2. Describe visual/statistical and probabilistic approaches to show how to analyze single-subject data.

3. Describe the strengths and limitations of these designs and methodologies.
4. Introduce the new probabilistic models for the analysis of single subject data, such as Bayesian Statistical Methods with C-statistics and Beta Distribution, and show how to perform them in a step-by-step approach.

Part II examines some areas of clinical practice or clinical research (mainly in the realm of communication disorders) where SSDs have been employed to evaluate treatment efficacy:

1. Treatment of anomia in aphasia (Section A);
2. Treatment of dysarthria (Section B);
3. General clinical and rehabilitation psychology (Section C);
4. Assessment of speech and hearing following cochlear implants (Section D); and
5. Training interventions for children with autism (Section E).

These five areas represent merely a sample of the many areas of clinical practice and research where SSDs are used. Although the authors are cognizant of the numerous areas of communication disorders and clinical psychology where single subject designs (SSDs) are applied, the reader is reminded that emphasis of this handbook is on methods of statistical analysis for SSDs. The small set of clinical examples described in Section II add a practical dimension to the statistical methods but do not represent the extent of clinical areas where utilization of SSDs can be found.

For each of the areas covered in Section II, actual clinical studies are described. Emphasis is given to the unique structure and constraints of the clinical scenarios to which SSDs are aptly suited. This is followed by hypothetical examples of clinical studies utilizing single subject designs. Illustrations are given on how to analyze the data for each example, visually and statistically, in determining the effect of intervention.

Although a fundamental working knowledge of elementary to intermediate statistics and basic research methods is essential for a thorough understanding of all the material, a large portion of the handbook can be read by those without a strong background in single subject research design. Parts of the book that illustrate methods of analysis in SSDs necessarily include some higher algebra and elementary differential calculus but this should not prevent the general reader from appreciating the greater portion of methods of analysis. Throughout the book, the authors highlight conceptual and procedural knowledge that can facilitate analytic methods in single subject designs. The question-and-answer format makes for a step-by-step approach—each procedure identifies the information and computa-

tions needed to solve a well-defined class of problems. This format gives users an easy way to answer specific questions about methodologies and designs and thus reinforce their knowledge. A great deal of attention is also given to linking the concepts described to the working formulae of specific statistical methods. To aid conceptual understanding, figures, tables, and graphs have been used to a greater extent than is typical of other statistics handbooks. These visual representations help confer a deeper level of understanding of the statistical methods for analyzing and interpreting single subject data.

It is the authors' hope that this book will benefit both students and clinical practitioners by offering a working knowledge of the principles of single subject research designs and various related data analysis techniques. Readers can expect a concise approach to a rich understanding of the concepts of single subject designs, delivered simply and effectively.

Acknowledgments

We would like to acknowledge all the hard working clinicians in the field who strive to improve their effectiveness by using a range of behavioral interventions in their everyday practice that are scientifically based and subject to empirical evaluation. Hopefully, the methods of data analysis discussed herein will be found to have many useful applications in evaluating treatment efficacy while advancing the quality of clinical decision making. We also thank our graduate assistants, in particular, Jamie Rumpf and Jane Emes for all their hard work and dedication in assisting us with the preparation of the manuscript.

Eike Satake
Vinoth Jagaroo
David. L. Maxwell

PART I

Theoretical Foundations and Statistical Methods of Single Subject Research: Most Frequently Asked Questions

SECTION A

Frequently Asked Questions

Question 1: What is Single-Subject Research?

- It refers to the study of a single subject over a period of time (or phases) to determine whether or not a given treatment (intervention) is effective in changing one's behavior or score. The most typically used single-subject research designs are as follows:

  1. The investigator obtains pretreatment measures (baseline, denoted by A) and then introduces an intervention (treatment, denoted by B). The investigator continues to measure the subject's scores after an intervention is introduced. Then, the investigator determines whether or not any evident change in the dependent variable from the baseline has occurred. (This design is called the A-B design.)

  2. In addition to the format of the A-B design, the investigator removes the intervention to determine if the subject's score returns to the baseline phase (A). (This design is called the A-B-A design.)

Question 2: What are the other names for Single-Subject Designs?

- Single-subject designs are also called (a) small-N designs, (b) N = 1 designs, (c) intensive designs, and (d) idiographic designs.

Question 3: What are philosophical and historical foundations of Single-Subject Designs?

- They are rooted in the work of B. F. Skinner and many other advocates of operant conditioning or applied behavioral analysis. Skinner stated: "Establish the behavior in which you are interested, submit the organism to a particular treatment, and look again at the behavior" (Skinner, 1953).

- In clinical-behavioral sciences, advocates of single subject designs have long argued that these designs often prove more useful than group designs concerned with classical hypothesis testing.

- Single subject designs provide expedient methods for evidence-based practice in general; hence, evidence generated therewith may lead to greater acceptance by the public and those influential in the creation of public policy (Robey et al., 1999).

Question 4: What are advantages of Single-Subject Designs?

- They are advantageous when only a few or a limited number of subjects are available for a study.
- They allow for better intrasubject control than group studies.
- They can help identify functional relationships between an independent variable and a dependent variable, something a typical case study does not allow.
- They offer capability for examination of both intersubject and intrasubject variability.
- They allow an investigator to correctly identify a confounding (extraneous) variable more easily than in group design.
- They are well adapted for meeting quality-assurance standards demanded by public and private health care agencies and organizations.
- They are applicable to a range of clinical scenarios in behavioral-health sciences. In clinical/counseling psychology, they have been described as "the best kept secret . . . " (Lundervold & Belwood, 2000).

Question 5: What are the major goals of Single-Subject Research?

- To gain precise control over the experimental conditions by eliminating extraneous variables.

- To establish a stable level of responding (baseline) before administering an intervention.
- To record the treated behavior within a given time period.
- To perform a visual and/or statistical/ probabilistic analysis of the data to determine the treatment outcome.

Question 6: What are limitations of Single-Subject Designs?

- A major concern about the single-subject design is external validity, that is, the result of one observation can accurately generalize to others or a target population. (It can be easily argued that such a lack of external validity may be corrected by replication.)

Assessing change with single-subject data is difficult because current statistical and non-statistical (visual approach) methods are unreliable and cannot control Type I and Type II errors effectively.

Question 7: What are the commonly used Single-Subject Designs?

1. *A-B Design:* The most basic of the small-N (time series) designs in which observations are made over a period of time to establish a baseline (A) prior to a treatment, for the subsequent comparison of retest data. Next, a treatment or intervention (B) is introduced and the investigator observes changes in the dependent variable to determine the effectiveness of the treatment.

2. *A-B-A Design:* A type of small-N time series design in which a baseline (A) condition is first established followed by a treatment (intervention) condition (B), and then finally by the withdrawal of the treatment condition, that is, return to baseline (A). It is also called a reversal design. The logic of the A-B-A design is as follows: If the treatment is effective, there exists some change (most likely a positive change) in the dependent variable after treatment is introduced, and there will be a return to the baseline condition when the treatment is withdrawn.

3. *A-B-A-B Design:* The most commonly used of the small-N time series designs. First, a baseline (A) phase is established. Second, treatment (B) is introduced. Third, treatment is withdrawn, that is, return to the baseline (A). Fourth, treatment (B) is reintroduced to assess its reliability. A variation of this design involves substituting an independent variable in the final B condition that is different from the first B condition. In effect, the A-B-A-B sequence involves the study of the treatment effect as it both precedes and follows a baseline phase. Clinically, the fourth phase of such a design is highly desirable as it avoids the negative consequences of the A-B-A experiment, which leaves subjects at the end of the study as they were in the beginning, namely, in a state comparable to their original baseline level of responding. A-B-A-B designs are also called replication designs.

4. *Alternating Treatment Design:* Two treatments, A and B, are alternated randomly as they are applied to a single subject. The results are examined to determine whether one of the two treatments is more effective than the other. It is also called a "between-series design."

5. *Reversal Design:* This design is similar to the ABA design with an important exception. During the third phase, instead of withdrawing treatment, a second form of intervention is applied and the effects of the two treatments are then compared. As usual, baseline measures are first recorded prior to a treatment. An intervention is then introduced that is followed in the next phase by a therapeutic reversal in intervention, namely, a different therapeutic intervention. For practical and ethical reasons, caution has to be exercised when using this particular design.

6. *Multiple-Baseline Design:* A small-N design that involve the application of a treatment to different baselines at different times. The main steps in the use of any multiple-baseline designs are as follows:
   a. Establish reliable and stable baselines on all behaviors selected for modification.
   b. Randomly select a behavior (or a subject or setting) for treatment while simultaneously observing an untreated behavior (or subject or setting).
   c. Randomly select another untreated baseline and introduce the experimental treatment.
   d. Continue until all baselines have been treated.
   e. Demonstrate treatment effectiveness by showing systematic modifications in performance across more than one baseline.

7. *Changing Criterion Design:* A variation of the small-N design. First, a series of behavioral criteria are established. A treatment plan is then introduced and its effectiveness is judged based on the extent to which the response level of the target behavior matches the present criteria.

Question 8: What are the advantages/disadvantages of each design?

Advantages	Limitations

A-B Design (Figure A–1)	
▨ Least complicated design and easy to implement.	▨ The lack of control of extraneous variables for determining treatment efficacy, that is, internal validity issue should be noted. Replication may correct the problem.

A-B-A Design (Figure A–2)	
▨ Affords greater experimental control by adding a second A.	▨ Difficult to interpret the follow-up data (a second A), after the treatment (B) is terminated. ▨ A possible ethical concern for some investigators relates to withholding treatment when a second baseline is used.

A-B-A-B Design (Figure A–3)	
▨ Allows for demonstrating the influence of the independent variable on two occasions. ▨ Clinically, the fourth phase B is highly desirable as it avoids the negative consequences of the A-B-A design that leave subjects at the end of the study as they were in the beginning—in a state comparable to their original baseline level of responding.	▨ Same ethical concern as described for the A-B-A design. A possible mitigating factor involves gaining more confidence in the design's potential efficacy by demonstrating its positive influence during a second treatment period.

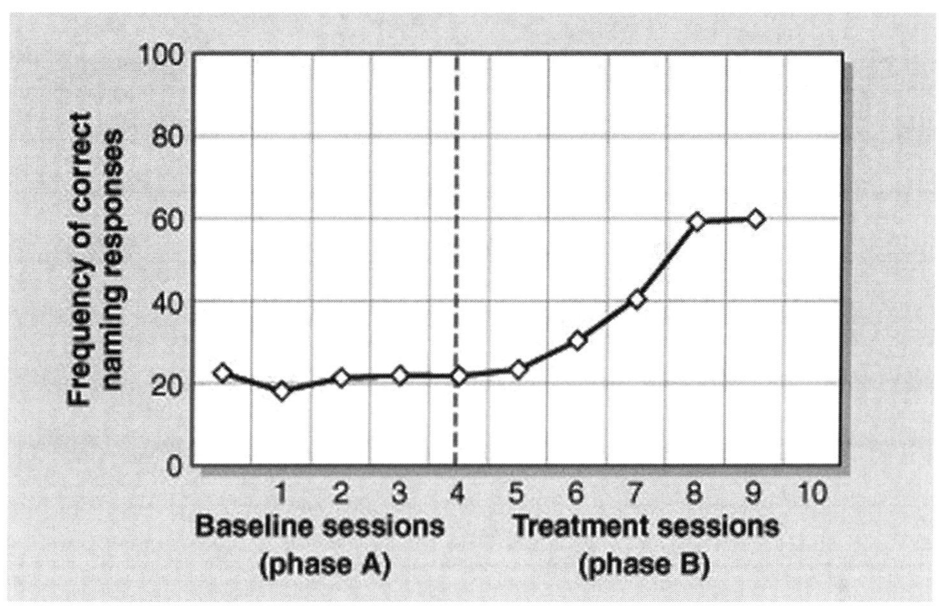

Figure A–1. Illustration of the A–B Design.

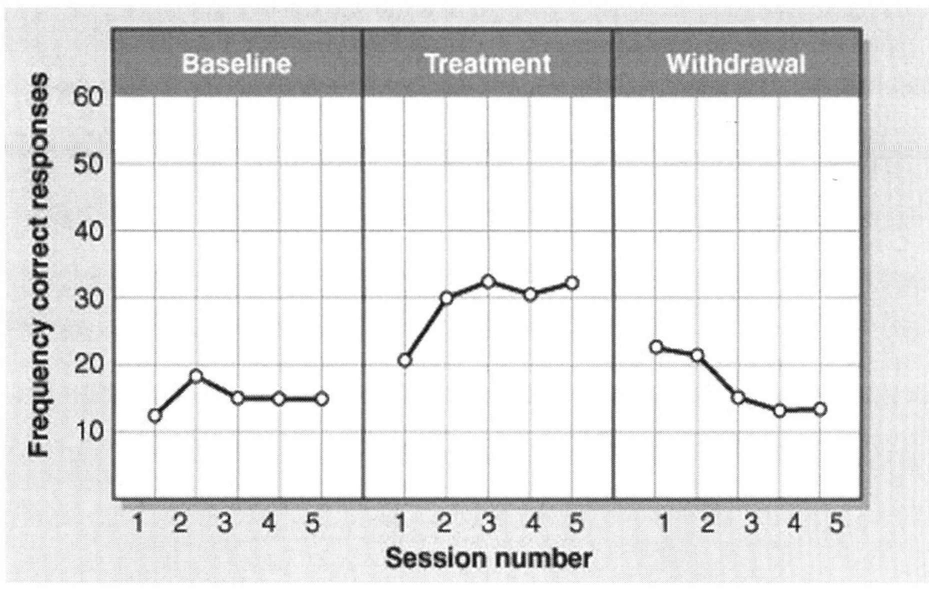

Figure A–2. Illustration of the A–B-A Design.

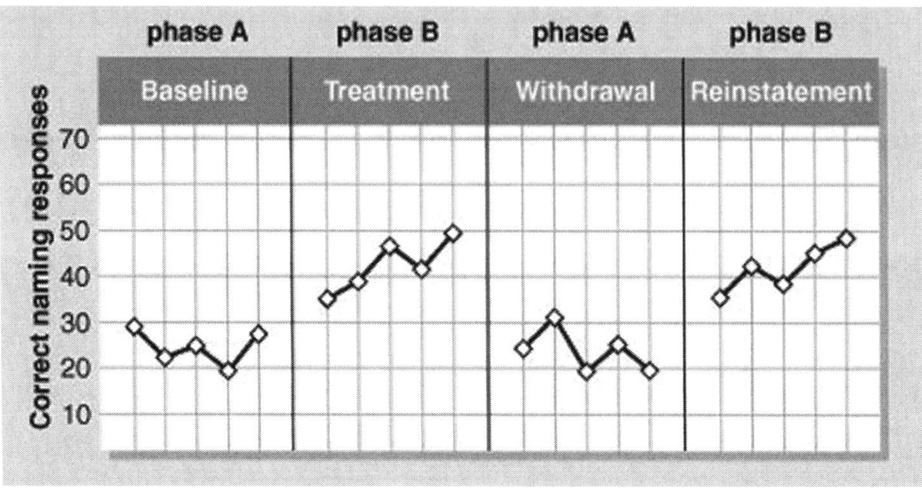

Figure A–3. Illustration of the A–B-A–B Design.

Advantages	Limitations

Alternating Treatments (Figure A-4)	
◼ Some type of treatment is always being used. ◼ Comparing differences between alternative treatments can assess their relative effectiveness.	◼ Can be associated with multiple-treatment interference effects, that is, the tendency of preceding treatments to make later treatments more or less effective. ◼ Can result from the order in which treatments are given or from the effects of one treatment carrying over to another.

Multiple-Baseline (Figure A-5)	
◼ Do not necessitate withdrawal of treatment to demonstrate treatment efficacy.	◼ Effects arising from treating the first behavior in a series might carry over and/or affect other behaviors under treatment. If this occurs, a true treatment effect would not be detected.

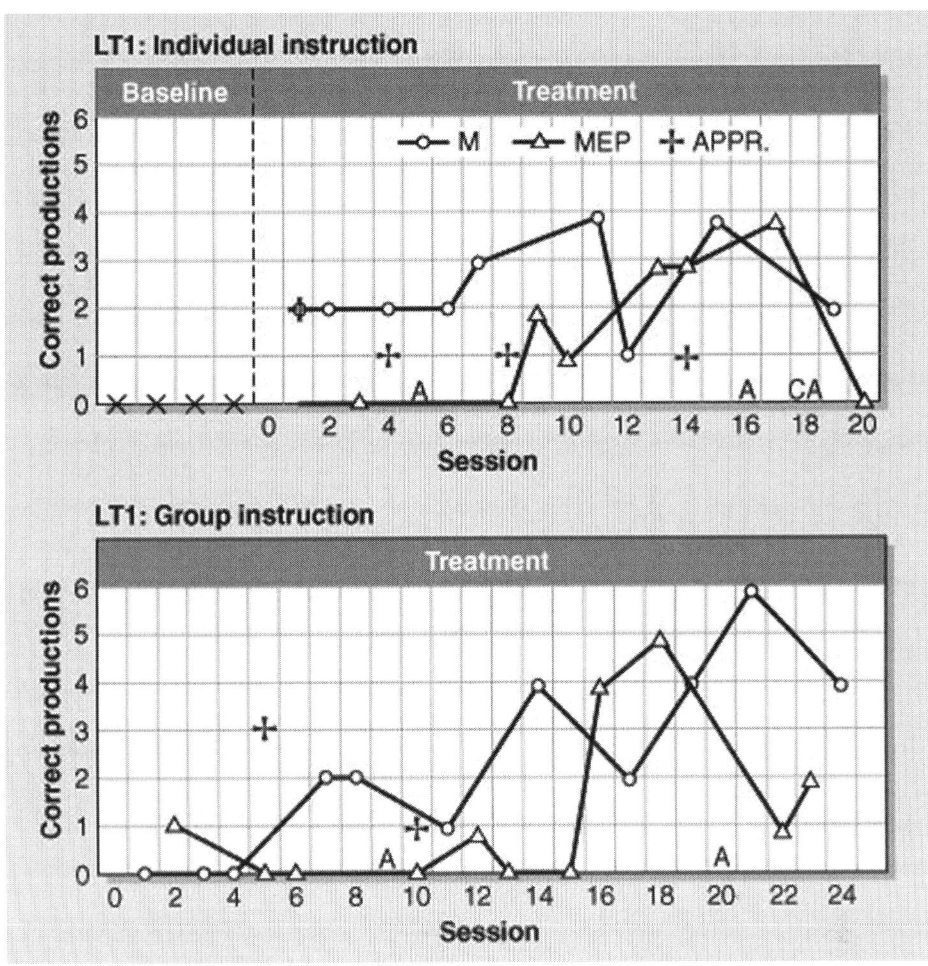

Figure A–4. Illustration of Alternating Treatments.

Advantages	Limitations
▪ Well suited for a variety of clinical applications, especially when an investigator wishes to monitor several treatments concurrently.	▪ Problems resulting from failure to achieve stable baselines prior to intervention. ▪ Large amount of time needed to collect data.

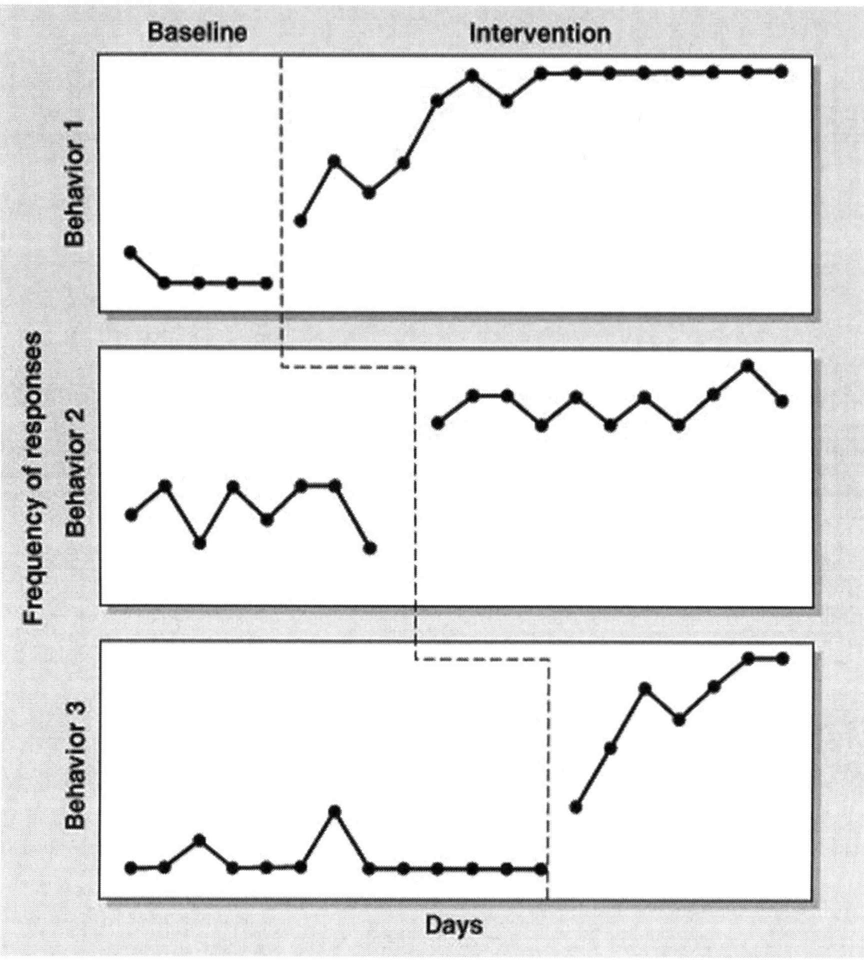

Figure A–5. Illustration of a Multiple-Baseline Design

Advantages	Limitations

Reversal (Figure A-6)	
▤ Gains power in illustrating the efficacy of a clinical intervention.	▤ Possibility of being unable to reverse some negative consequences associated with the effort to demonstrate experimental control over the targeted behavior. Thus, for practical and ethical reasons, caution should be exercised in the use of this design.

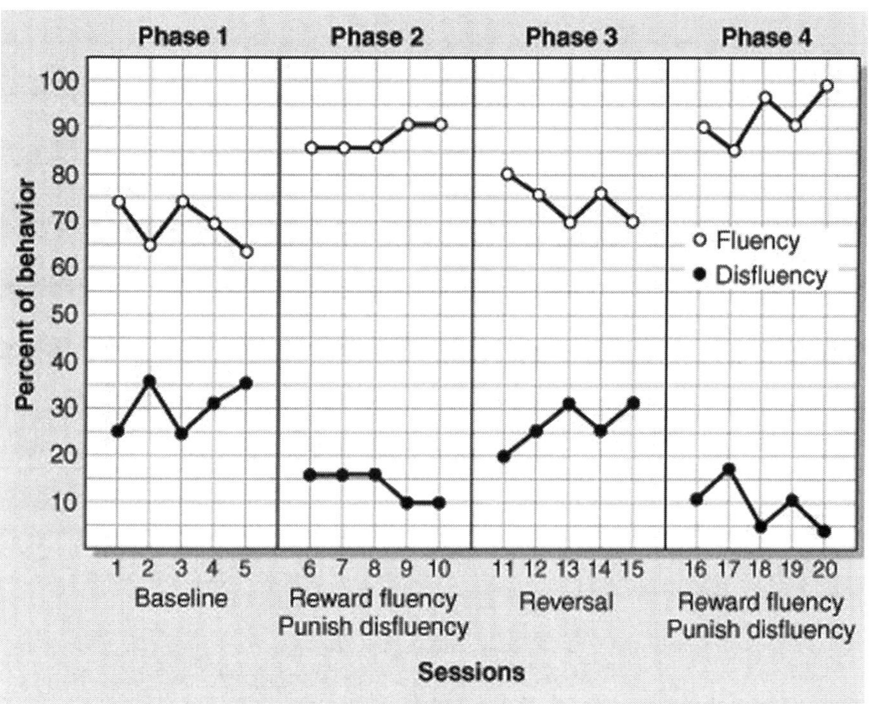

Figure A–6. Illustration of a Reversal Design (for treating stuttering and hypothetical results). The contingencies of phase 2 are reversed in phase 3. In phase 4, the phase 2 contingencies are reinstated.

Advantages	Limitations

Changing Criterion Design	
▩ Has many useful applications to clinical or applied settings in which random assignment of individuals to treatment conditions is impractical or impossible to achieve.	▩ Falls short of meeting the randomization requirement of true experiments.

Question 9: How do we evaluate treatment efficacy in Single-Subject Research?

Visual/Graphical Methods

1. Split-Middle
2. Celeration Line
3. Two Standard Deviation Rule
4. Frequency Histogram
5. Bar Graph

Strengths	**Limitations**
■ All data are presented as a single source so that it is less time-consuming and less complex when analyzing and interpreting the results. ■ Uses more direct descriptive approaches to describe the population parameter (a single subject) in which one has all information, whereas inferential statistics are used to make predictions about an entire population based on representative samples of behavior.	■ Tends to produce a low level of agreement among raters concerning the research result. ■ Lack of universally accepted decision criteria in detecting a change. ■ Excessive risk of a Type I error (no actual change but rated as showing a treatment effect) especially when the number of sample data points is small. ■ Less statistical power, that is, more Type II error (actual change but rated as showing no treatment effect) may be committed when the number of sample data points is small.

Statistical Methods

Inferential
1. *t*-test
2. ANOVA
3. Mann-Whitney U test
4. Regression

Time Series
1. Moving Average
2. Interrupted time-series analysis (ITSA)
3. A new interrupted time-series analysis (ITSACORR)
4. The C-statistic

Probabilistic
1. Binomial tests
2. Bayesian analysis with C-statistic (Jones, 2003)
3. Bayesian analysis with beta probability (Maxwell & Satake, 2006)

Nonparametric
1. Chi-Square test

Strengths	**Limitations**
▣ It is reliable and when its assumptions (normality, independence, and homogeneity or variances) are met, it maintains Type I error at the satisfactory level. ▣ It can detect small but consistent treatment effects. ▣ In contrast to visual approaches, it produces consistent and more scientific results across data analysis.	▣ The results of a hypothesis test depend on both effect size and sample size in the study. Small effects that may be statistically significant may have very little practical or clinical significance. ▣ An inappropriate conclusion is often associated with rejecting a null hypothesis. ▣ Parametric assumptions must be satisfied in order to obtain an accurate result. ▣ When data values are positively autocorrelated (each value is more similar to its preceding value than to the mean), observations are more similar to each other. This leads to artificial deflation of error variances and inflation of a t and/or F value. Hence, it increases the probability of making a Type I error. ▣ Negatively autocorrelated data values (each value is less similar to its preceding value than to the mean) are more dissimilar to each other than would occur by chance. This leads to artificial inflation of error variance and deflation of a t and/or F value. Hence, it increases the probability of making a Type II error. ▣ When we use regression analysis, many actual data points that are further away from the central zone will be dropped and removed from the final analysis. It may produce an inaccurate result especially when the number of sample data points are small. ▣ When we use moving average time-series analysis, moving average values can be extremely inconsistent and discrepant with the actual trend of existing data set, that is, the mean (or median) value neglects the true value of the measure of dispersion. It must be calculated on the actual data values, not the average values, to increase the accuracy of the results.

Question 10: In general, how do we analyze single-subject data visually (i.e., how do we detect a change of one's response by using the visual/graphical approach)?

- To determine the cause of one's change, a horizontal stable baseline is a desired characteristic in single-subject research.
- *Phase Length:* a minimum of at least three consecutive observations should be used for purposes of plotting data points during each phase of the experiment. As far as possible, the baseline phase should continue until stability in the targeted behavior has been established.
- *Change one variable at a time:* when moving from one phase to another, only one independent variable should be altered so that its influence can be observed and recorded independent of any other influence.
- *Level:* refers to the magnitude of the data points on a graph. Typically, the change of the y-intercept indicates the level change between baseline phase (A) and intervention phase (B). Two aspects to examine include the level stability and level change of data.
  a. *Level Stability:* the range of the data point value determines level stability within a particular phase of the experiment regardless of whether it is a baseline phase or treatment phase. As a general guide, if 80% to 90% of the data points of a condition fall within a 15% range of the mean level of all data point values of a condition, they are considered to be level stable (Tawney & Gast, 1984).
  b. *Level Change:* to determine the change in the level of the dependent variable between the baseline and treatment phases of an experiment, compare the last data point of the baseline phase with the first data point of the treatment phase. Only adjacent phases can serve as valid comparisons of data points. Generally, the sooner a change in response level is observed following the introduction of treatment and the greater its magnitude in relation to baseline, the more confidence we can have in the treatment effect. It is also possible to identify the degree of level change within a particular phase. A simple way to accomplish this is to (a) identify the first and last data points of a phase, (b) subtract the smaller of the values from the larger, and (c) observe whether the change in level is in a positive or negative direction based on the treatment objectives (Tawney & Gast, 1984).
- *Trend:* in general, it refers to the slope (rate of change) of the data points on a graph. The data points can be said to be accelerating (increasing with respect to their ordinate values), decelerating (decreasing with respect to their ordinate values), or may show zero slope (data points are level with abscissa). Figure A–7 illustrates these three trend characteristics found in single-subject data.
- However, should the slopes of the data points in adjacent phases move in the same direction, it is difficult to detect a treatment effect under such circumstances. This is because such a change simply may be due to extraneous variables such as maturation, history, and the like.
- Furthermore, should the data points illustrate a large degree of fluctuation

Three Different Trend Characteristics

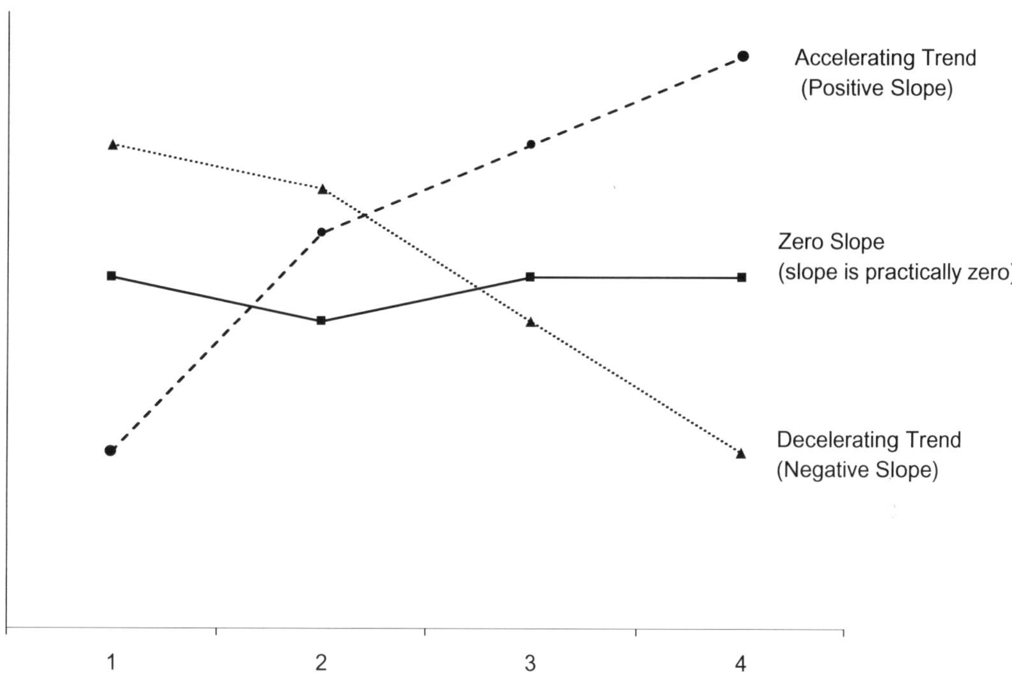

Figure A–7. Three different trend characteristics.

during the baseline phase, the number of trials during this phase should be increased until either (1) a stable response rate is demonstrated, that is, response rate = $\frac{response\ frequency}{time}$, or (2) the trend of the direction of behavior of interest is opposite to that of the intended treatment effect.

Question 11: How do we determine "Changes in Level" and "Changes in Trend" graphically?

See Figure A–8.

Question 12: What is a Celeration Line?

■ To estimate the slope of the trend, the most commonly used visual approach is to draw a straight line that most closely approximates the majority of the data points in a series. Such a line is called a celeration line. The procedures for obtaining a celeration line are identical to those for obtaining a split-middle line except that means are used instead of medians. The instructions of drawing such a line for a hypothetical series of data points are shown in Figure A 9 and described below.

How do we know "Change in Level" and "Change in Trend" graphically?

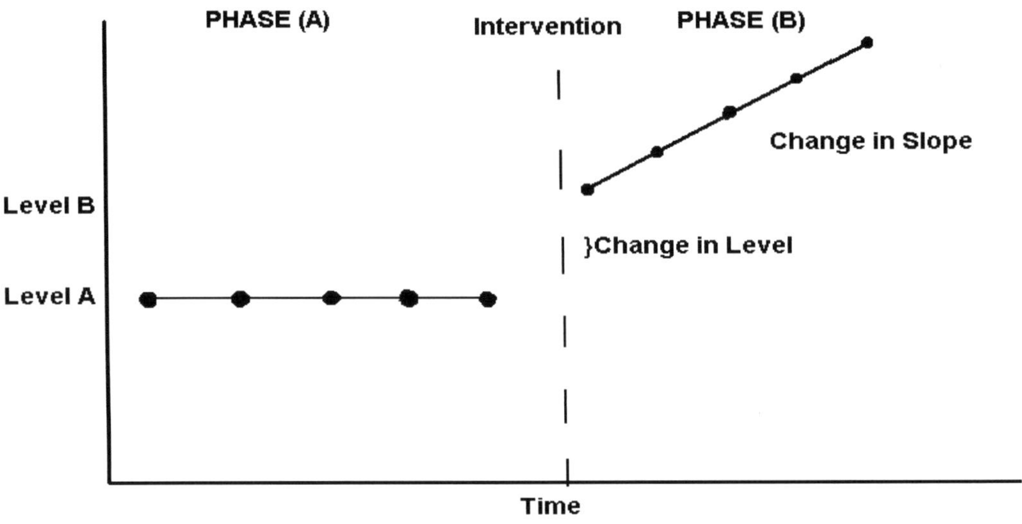

Figure A–8. Illustration of "Changes in slope" and "Changes in Level" in A–B design.

How to Draw a Celeration Line

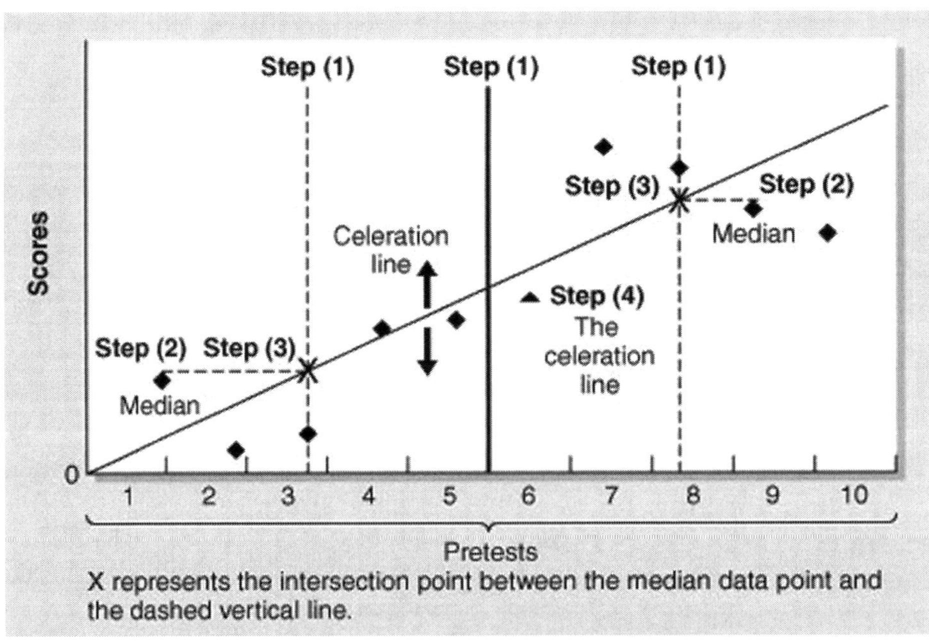

Figure A–9. Illustration of a Celeration Line.

Instructions for Drawing a Celeration Line (Figure A-9)

X represents the intersection point between the median data point and the dashed vertical line.

Step 1. Count the total number of data points in the baseline phase (pretest 1 to pretest 10) and divide this number so that half fall on one side of a solid vertical line and the remaining half fall on the other side. As can be seen, the solid line falls directly in the center of the graph. Next, draw a second dashed vertical line on each side of the solid vertical line that again divides the data points in half.

Step 2. Identify the median score for the data distribution on each side of the solid vertical line. The median is the middle value of the data points with respect to their magnitude.

Step 3. Draw a dashed horizontal line through the median data point on each side of the solid vertical line so it intersects the dashed vertical lines.

Step 4. Draw a straight solid line by connecting the two points of intersection (denoted by *X*) passing through the solid vertical line. This final step completes the construction of the celeration line. In this case, we can visually determine that the trend of the data points is accelerating. However, based on such a visual analysis alone, we cannot determine the *rate of change*— how fast the dependent variable changes over time. This determination can only be made by the use of statistical methods that are beyond the scope of the present chapter.

Question 13: What is the Two Standard Deviation Method? (a.k.a. a 2 SD method)

- A methodfor determining whether or not the level of change observed in a graph is a reliable change due to a treatment effect, that is., significantly different from the baseline phase.
- Instructions for using a two standard deviation method are shown in Figure A-10 and described below.

Instructions for Using a 2 Standard Deviation Method (Figure A-10)

1. Plot the data points for a baseline phase (A). Then compute the mean ($\bar{x}$) and standard deviation (SD) of the baseline data values.
2. Draw a 2 SD confidence interval around $\bar{x}$ and observe whether, during a treatment phase (B), at least two successive data points fall outside a two SD interval. If they do, a significant change has occurred due to a treatment. As seen in Figure A-10, a significant change has occurred since the last 3 treatment days fell outside the 2 SD interval.

Question 14: What is the significance of the use of statistical analysis in Single-Subject Research?

- Investigators need to know the likelihood of the change due to either random chance or a true treatment

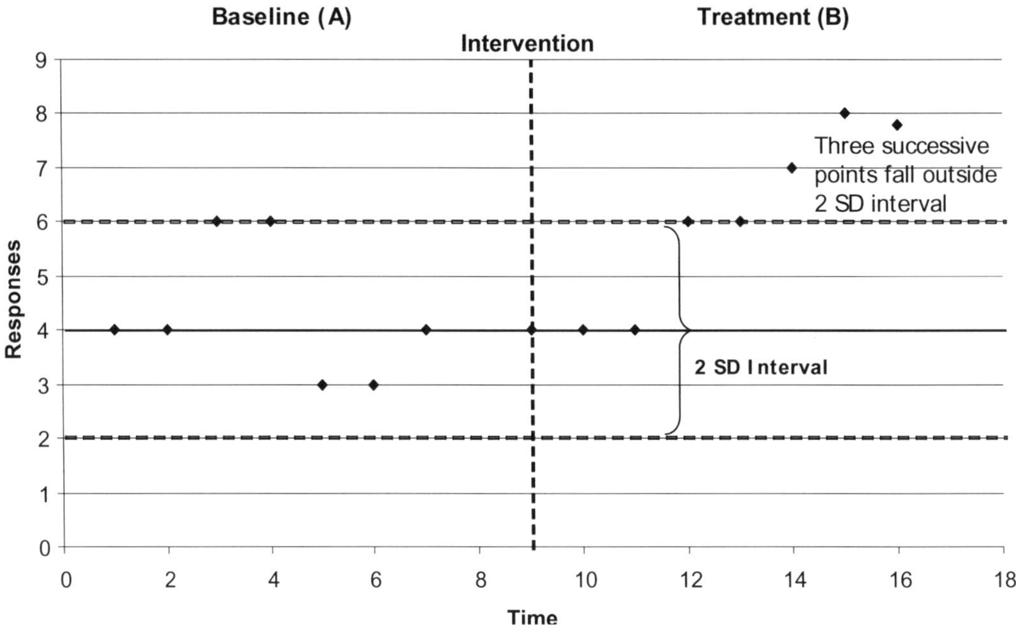

Figure A–10. Illustration of a Two Standard Deviation method.

effect in many cases, that is, "what is the probability that the successful outcome derived from a particular study was the result of chance or a true treatment effect?" This question cannot be answered by the visual approach alone but it can be answered by the use of various appropriate statistical analyses.

Question 15: Statistically, how do we control error variance (due to chance)?

- With group-designs, error variance (V_e) is controlled experimentally (by means of randomization).
- With single-subject designs, error variance (V_e) is controlled using

replication and as much as possible experimentally (see Question 16 below).

Question 16: What do we mean by "experimentally"?

- Investigators must identify the factor(s) affecting one's behavior and the confounding factor(s), other than treatment through therapy, counseling, and so forth.
- Using subjects as their own controls, comparing a statistical difference between baseline to intervention time periods.
- Replication across subjects is also used in single-subject research to enhance control.

Question 17: What are the general procedures of the classical statistical methods in Single-Subject Research?

- If autocorrelation, denoted by r, (Pearson correlation coefficient involving serial dependency in a temporally order sequence of data points) is not statistically significant (or it is believed to be nonsignificant visually), you may proceed with a t-test, ANOVA, or the nonparametric Mann-Whitney U test.

Question 18: What is a time series and how do we evaluate data values?

- Time-series analysis is about whether there is an evident "trend" in the sequential measurements.
- Trend is evaluated by two components: slope (evaluated visually by the time series graph) and magnitude (y-intercept) evaluated using the C-statistic).
- The most commonly used methods are moving average (a series of the mean of successive data point values), interrupted time-series analysis (autocorrelational time series), and a revised interrupted time-series analysis (improved version of interrupted time-series analysis)

Question 19: What are the limitations of time-series analysis?

- Moving average values can be extremely inconsistent (a greater degree of fluctuation) with the actual trend of real existing data set, that is, the mean (or median) value of lag-1 (or 2, 3, etc. For further detail, please refer to Question 25.) neglects the true value of measure of dispersion. It must be calculated on the actual data values, not the average values, to increase the accuracy of observation.

Question 20: What is the limitation of the regressional/correlational method?

- To find a line of best fit, many actual data points (that are further away from the central zone) will be dropped and removed from the final analysis.

Question 21: How do we maintain the power of a statistical test in Single-Subject Research?

- In many cases, the quality and form of the data would suggest that you use a more conservative approach (if one of the parametric assumptions is violated, i.e., normality, independence, and homogeneity of variances) with the nonparametric test for data analysis.
- The disadvantage of the use of the nonparametric test is less power in detecting a significant change between the phases, that is to say, you may risk failing to reject a null hypothesis when differences between phases (variables) are, in fact, unlikely to have occurred by chance alone.
- You can still choose to perform the parametric methods, regardless of the

violation of parametric assumptions. With that decision, the risk is that you will reject the null hypothesis when the differences were actually the result of peculiarities in the data rather than differences in the treatment.

- The best approach is to use both visual and statistical (including probabilistical) methods when analyzing single-subject data values. Also, this statistical analysis is exclusively designed for determining whether or not a change is "statistically significant" and does not address whether or not the change is "clinically or theoretically significant."

Question 22: What is the C-statistic?

- It is one of the simplest ways to calculate the change of "slope of the baseline" and "slope of the intervention period."
- A primary advantage of the C-statistic for a single-subject data series is that it requires a fewer number of datapoints. As few as eight data points per phase can be employed with little loss of power to detect a change of slope and trend. (Jones, 2003)

Question 23: How do we calculate C?

- The value of C is given by:

$$C = 1 - \frac{\sum_{t=1}^{n-1}(x_t - x_{t+1})^2}{2 \cdot \sum_{t=1}^{n}(x_t - \bar{x})^2}$$

where x_i = the ith data point in the combined stream of n data points in phases A and B

$\bar{x}$ = overall mean

- The ratio of C to its standard deviation (SD) gives a Z value, which provides the probability value of assessing the tenability of the null hypothesis.

$$Z = \frac{C}{SD} \quad \text{where SD} = \sqrt{\frac{n-2}{(n-1) \cdot (n+1)}}$$

Question 24: What is the rationale behind the C-statistic in actual clinical practice?

- The logic of the C-statistic for application in actual clinical practice is (1) continue baseline measures until there is no evident random variation (almost stable horizontally); and (2) after a treatment is given, you observe whether or not data points in the treatment phase become significantly different from data points in baseline phase based on a p-value.

Question 25: What is the difference between time series with the C-statistic and time series with autocorrelation?

- In essence, autocorrelation is a form of Pearson's product moment correlation coefficient (r). The most widely used autocorrelation in single-subject research is called "Lag-1," that is, a correlation of each data point with the immediately following observed point in the series. It calculates the statistical trend of data within each of the phases of a design.

■ In the C-statistic, an analysis of each phase is conducted separately and then the analysis of the outcome of the two phases are combined, that is., baseline analysis, treatment analysis, and both baseline and treatment analysis.

Question 26: How do we conduct a Chi-square test in a Single-Subject Design?

■ Categorize "desired" outcomes (falls at or above the celeration/split-middle line) and "undesired" outcomes (falls below the celeration/split-middle line) using either a celeration or split-middle line for a 2×2 contingency table analysis. This is shown in Figure A–11 below in an A-B design.

■ The basic steps for the method can be summarized as follows.
   1. Identify whether or not there is evident change (increase or decrease) in the baseline phase.
   2. Extend the celeration (or split-middle) line through the treatment phase.
   3. The two columns in the first row for the analysis are the number of points in the baseline data that are at or above the celeration line (or split-middle line), called "Desired," and the number of data points that are below the line, called "Undesired."
   4. Comparable data for the treatment phase provide the second row for the analysis.

Illustration of a two by two Chi-Square Table

	Desired	Undesired	Subtotal
Baseline			
Treatment			
Subtotal			Total Points

Figure A–11. Illustration of a two-by-two Chi-square table.

5. Calculate an observed χ^2 value and conclude it.

H_o: No change H_a: Evident Change

Observed χ^2 value $= \sum \dfrac{(O-E)^2}{E}$

with degrees of freedom $=$
$(Row-1) \bullet (Column-1)$
$O =$ number of data points
$E =$ expected number of data points

$$= \dfrac{(Row\ Subtotal) \bullet (Column\ Subtotal)}{Grand\ Total}$$

for an appropriate category

Question 27: What is a binomial expansion test and how is it performed?

- A binomial test is focused on the consistency of whatever differences may occur whereas a t-test, ANOVA, and Mann-Whitney U test focus on "how much" difference exists between the phases. The outcome of the binomial analysis is a direct probability of occurrence of a particular event of interest.
- To calculate the binomial probability, we need (a) number of trials, and (b) number of "successful" outcomes (it means "how many" data points meet your criteria). Then, we calculate it as follows:

P (k successes in n trials) $=$

$$_nC_k \bullet p^k \bullet (1-p)^{n-k}$$

where $_nC_k =$ number of different arrangements can be made in selecting k successes from a total of n trials,

$$_nC_k = \dfrac{n!}{k! \bullet (n-k)!}$$

$n!$ represents (n factorial) the product of n consecutive integers from n to 1.

$P =$ probability of a success

Question 28: In a binomial analysis, how do we state hypotheses?

- The null hypothesis (H_o) states that a population proportion in the baseline phase (A), denoted by π_b, is equal to the population proportion in the intervention phase (B), denoted by π_i. Symbolically it is written as follows:

H_o: $\pi_b = \pi_i$ (No evident change)
H_a: $\pi_b \neq \pi_i$: (Evident change)

- Count the number of data points that fall below the celeration (or split-middle) line, and we write:

$\hat{\pi}_b =$
$$\dfrac{(number\ of\ data\ points\ falling\ below\ the\ line)}{total\ number\ of\ data\ points}$$
(baseline)

$\hat{\pi}_i =$
$$\dfrac{(number\ of\ data\ points\ falling\ below\ the\ line)}{total\ number\ of\ data\ points}$$
(intervention)

where $\hat{\pi}_b$ and $\hat{\pi}_i$ are called "a point estimate" for π_b and π_i, respectively.

- Cohen (1988) recommends that the test of H_o should be rewritten as:

$$H_o: \varnothing_b = \varnothing_i$$
$$where\ \hat{\varnothing}_b = 2\,arc\,sin\sqrt{\hat{\pi}_t}$$

Using the critical value given by Cohen (1988), we may draw a conclusion whether or not evident change occurred.

Question 29: Are there any new developments in statistical methods for Single-Subject Designs?

■ We have successfully implemented a so-called "Bayesian Probabilistic Approach" with C-statistics (Jones, 2003) and/or Beta Distribution (Maxwell & Satake, 2006) into the single-subject designs. Using this approach, we do not have to be concerned about the usual parametric assumptions, such as "Normality," "Independence," and "Homogeneity of Variances."

Question 30: What is Bayesian analysis?

■ A mathematical basis for determining the degree to which a prior belief corresponds with the actual facts of subse-quent observations. Statistically, a formula of calculating the inverse conditional probability of an event, P (A given B), from the conditional probability of an-other event, P (B given A) and the unconditional probability of the event $P(A)$.

■ First described in 1763 by an English clergyman, Thomas Bayes, the Bayesian method provides a mathematical basis for expressing one's beliefs in the language of probability prior to collect-ing data. Such a statement, called the prior probability, is akin to the research hypothesis (or alternate hypothesis) with the additional requirement of including a numerical or quantitative estimate or "bet" reflecting the degree of belief about a predicted result. The next step is to derive a data probability based on the sample of data actually collected. The data probability can be regarded as the conditional credibility of a particular view pending the calculation of a posterior probability. The latter probability, reflecting the updated credibility of an original opinion or viewpoint, is derived from a mathematical combination of the prior and data probabilities.

Question 31: How does Bayesian analysis work?

■ Prior Probability (one's subjective belief) → New Data → Combined New Data with Prior Probability → Update Prior Probability → Posterior Probability (or a new prior probability) → New Data → Combined New Data with New Prior Probability → Update New Prior Probability → New Posterior Probability (or a new prior probability).

Keep repeating this cycle to derive the maximum likelihood of a particular event of your interest. This cumulative process provides a guide for changing existing one's belief as new evidence emerges.

Question 32: What is the rationale behind Bayesian analysis?

■ In a clinical setting, for instance, an investigator needs to evaluate the appropriate time/situation for providing a particular treatment to prevent them from further illness or dysfunction. In order to accomplish this task, what the invest-igator needs is a study design that is continuous and cumulative. The sta-tistical method called the Bayesian approach fulfills this goal. In the Bayesian view, the likelihood of the occurrence of the second data value is contingent on the occurrence of the first data value, symbolically we write P second data given that first data has already been observed. In short, the approach allows for collecting data prospectively.

- The ideal statistical model is a mixture of time-series analysis and cumulative probabilistic model. Bayesian analysis rests on a premise that the probability of a particular outcome on a particular day is contingent on the fact that all other outcomes in the preceding stages have already been observed.

Question 33: What are the differences between the classical statistical approach and the Bayesian probabilistic approach?

- A table comparing classical statistics to the Bayesian approach in hypothesis testing is illustrated in Table A–1.
- This table also summarizes the main differences between the two approaches.

Question 34: What is Bayesian analysis with C-statistic?

- Jones (2003) invented a method to test the hypothesis of randomness (evident change or not) of baseline + treatment

phases by means of Bayesian analysis. Tables A–2, A–3, and A–4 illustrate step-by-step procedures for this method of hypothesis testing.

Step 1: Calculate a *p*-value from baseline + treatment phase

Step 2: First replication: Calculate a new likelihood, a *p*-value of $z = \dfrac{C}{SD}$ again using a set of new data values (baseline + treatment).

Step 3: Second replication: Calculate a new likelihood, a *p*-value of $z = \dfrac{C}{SD}$ once again using a set of new data values (baseline + treatment), and so on. Keep repeating the procedure and we would eventually obtain the maximum likelihood posterior prob-ability of H_o and H_a. Murphy (2000) stated that the essence of the Bayesian approach is a mathematical rule to guide the change of existing belief when there is new evidence, instead of any one study serving a "stand-alone" role, each new set of observations of a study is conceptualized as a tool for modifying the prior belief.

Question 35: What is the Bayesian analysis with beta probabilities?

- Maxwell and Satake (2006) formulated and applied an alternative method using a probability distribution called a "beta distribution." It can be used for updating one's prior belief to eventually allow for derivation of the maximum likelihood of *p*-value. This can be accomplished by the replication of measurements. (For further details, see Appendix.)

Table A–1. Classical versus Bayesian Statistics

Sources	*Classical Statistics*	*Bayesian Statistics*
Number of hypotheses	Only two (null and alternative) hypotheses can be stated each time	Allowed to have two or more hypotheses at one time
Hypothesized values in initial hypothesis	More objective, views, or well-defined previous knowledge	Researcher is free to express subjective views from previous experience
Data Analysis	Normal Z, t, or F distributions	Beta Distribution with Gamma function
Assumptions of data analysis	1. Independence 2. Homogeneity of Variances	None
Type of conclusion derived	Rejection or nonrejection of null hypothesis. The hypothesis rejected is totally disregarded. No specific value of a true population parameter derived.	None of the hypotheses disregarded. Researcher estimates the credibility of each hypothesized value and derives the maximum likelihood of a true population parameter.
ANOVA	Researcher determines whether or not there are treatment effects on dependent variable(s). Significant or not.	Researcher considers how much each parameter (treatment effect) affects dependent variable(s); measures the strength of each treatment. Specific values that represent the degree of strength are derived.
ANOVA model selection	Trial and Error	The most powerful and suitable model can be found. How accurately does each model predict a future value?
MANOVA and ANOVA	Trial and Error	Same as above

Table A–2. Initial Calculation Procedures of Bayesian Analysis with a C-Statistic

Hypotheses	Prior Probability	Likelihood	Data Probability Prior Likelihood	Posterior Probability
H_o: No evident change (Random)	.5	p	$.5p$	$\dfrac{.5p}{\Sigma(sum)} = a$
H_a: Evident change (Not Random)	.5 Not having any substantial knowledge about the matter, it is recommended that the series start with equal prior probabilities (i.e., 50%-50%)	$1 - p$ p is derived from a normal obtained Z score, i.e., $Z = \dfrac{C}{SD}$	$.5(1 - p)$ $\Sigma(sum) =$ $.5p + .5(1 - p)$	$\dfrac{.5(1 - p)}{\Sigma(sum)} = 1 - a$ $\dfrac{Posterior\ Data}{\Sigma(sum)}$

Table A–3. Calculation Procedure in the First Replication Stage

Hypotheses	Prior	Likelihood	Data Prior × Likelihood	Probability
H_o: No evident change (Random)	a	p'	ap'	$\dfrac{ap'}{\Sigma(sum)} = b$
H_a: Evident change (Not Random)	$1 - a$	$1 - p'$	$(1 - a) \bullet (1 - p')$	$\dfrac{(1 - a) \bullet (1 - p')}{\Sigma(sum)} = 1 - b$
	Note that prior of the 1st replication is equal to posterior of the preceding series.	$p' = ap'$ value of the 1st replication, using $Z = \dfrac{C}{SD}$	$\Sigma(sum) = ap' +$ $(1 - a)(1 - p')$	$\dfrac{Data}{\Sigma(sum)}$

Table A–4. Calculation Procedure in the Second Replication

Hypotheses	Prior	Likelihood	Data Prior × Likelihood	Posterior
H_o: No evident change (Random)	b	p''	bp''	$\dfrac{bp''}{\Sigma(sum)} = C$
H_a: Evident change (Not Random)	$1 - b$	$1 - p''$	$(1 - b)\bullet(1 - p'')$	$\dfrac{(1 - b)\bullet(1 - p'')}{\Sigma(sum)} = 1 - C$
	Again, note that the prior probability of the 2nd replication is equal to the posterior probability of the 1st replication.	$p'' = ap''$ value of the 2nd replication, using $Z = \dfrac{C}{SD}$	$\Sigma(sum) = bp'' + (1 - b)(1 - p'')$	$\dfrac{Data}{\Sigma(sum)}$

Steps for conducting the Bayesian analysis with beta probablities

H_o: No evident change, H_a: Evident change, absence of assumptions of the classical parametric statistics.

Let us define:
- π = a point estimate (subjective or objective) of the binomial experiment
- n = sample size
- x = number of observations having a particular characteristic we are investigating

Then, the prior distribution of "Beta" may be written as follows:

$$f(\pi) = \frac{(a+b-1)!}{(a-1)!(b-1)!}\bullet \pi^{a-1}\bullet(1-\pi)^{b-1}$$

where μ' (1st prior mean) and σ'^2 (1st prior variance) are calculated as:

$$\mu' = \frac{a}{a+b}, \quad \sigma'^2 = \frac{\mu'\bullet(1-\mu')}{a+b+1}$$

Note that a and b are two non-negative integer parameters for π and the purpose of such constants is to simply adjust the beta curve in such a way that the area under the curve equals 100%, thereby making the function a probability distribution. The shape of the curve is adjusted by the exponents for π and $1 - \pi$. We can compute a and b algebraically as follows.

$$a = \mu' \bullet \left[\frac{\mu' \bullet (1-\mu')}{\sigma'^2} - 1 \right]$$

$$b = (1-\mu') \bullet \left[\frac{\mu' \bullet (1-\mu')}{\sigma'^2} - 1 \right]$$

The data values are assumed to satisfy the binomial distribution, such that for the true value of π the probability of the data can be found.

Data Probability =

$$f\langle x|\pi \rangle = \frac{n!}{x!(n-x)!} \bullet \pi^x \bullet (1-\pi)^{n-x}$$

$f\langle x|\pi \rangle$ means $f(x$ given $\pi)$

Next, we combine the prior probability and data probability together by Bayes' rule to derive the posterior probability:

$$f\langle \pi|x \rangle =$$

$$\frac{(n+a+b-1)!}{(x+a-1)!(n-x+b-1)!} \bullet \pi^{x+a-1} \bullet (1-\pi)^{n-x+b-1}$$

which is a beta distribution with parameters x+a and n−x+b. The posterior mean μ'' and variance σ''^2 can be computed as

$$\mu'' = \frac{x+a}{n+a+b} \qquad \sigma''^2 = \frac{\mu'' \bullet (1-\mu'')}{n+a+b+1}$$

Keep repeating this process by using the statistical software packages like MINITAB, SPSS, etc., we would again be able to derive the maximum likelihood *p*-value of a particular event of interest. One of the major advantages of this approach over others is that, for reasonably large exponents, the beta distribution can be approximated by the normal distribution and Bayesian probability intervals for π, regardless of n, can be easily found from $\mu \pm z_{\alpha/2} \bullet \sigma$.

Even when the beta curve is not entirely symmetric, the normal approximation is still quite good. As Iversen (1984) stated " . . . the reason Bayesian inference is so much more natural is that it is more closely geared to the research process itself than is classical inference. The research problem starts with an initial uncertainty about one or more parameters, data are collected in order to increase our information about the parameters, and in light of the new information, the initial uncertainty has been reduced."

Question 36: What is the Bayes factor and how do we interpret the test results with the Bayes factor?

■ In recent years, there has been growing awareness of and interest in the Bayesian approach as an alternative to the *p*-value approach and its applications to various clinical and research questions. The *p*-value approach has been criticized by many researchers over several years, largely due to (a) misinterpretation, of its meaning, (b) arbitrariness and use of $p = 0.05$ or 0.01 criteria for purposes of statistical significance testing, and (c) the *p*-value method is not an "Evidence-based" method. More specifically, contrary to what most clinical practitioners believe, *p*-values are conditional probabilities and calculated on the assumption that the null hypothesis (H_o) is true." Symbolically, the *p*-values are expressed as P (Data | H_o is true). More specifically, a typical *p*-value users tend to commit a crucial error, called "transposition of conditional fallacy," in which p (Data | H_o is true) is mistaken for P (H_o is true | Data). Basically, what clinical practitioners want to derive is the latter conditional probability (the inverse of the p-value, i.e., p (H_o is true | Data)), only the latter probability indicates evidential strength for the null hypothesis (H_o) versus the research hypothesis (H_A) after actual data are observed. Mathematically, this can be written as follows:

$$[P (H_o \text{ is true} | \text{Data})/ P (H_A \text{ is true} | \text{Data})]$$
$$= [P (H_o \text{ is true})/ P (H_A \text{ is true})] \times \lambda$$
$$\text{where } \lambda = \text{Bayes Factor} =$$
$$[P (\text{Data} | H_o \text{ is true})/ P (\text{Data} | (H_A \text{ is true})]$$

Simply, from the left to the right, we can also express it as follows:

$$\text{Posterior odds} =$$
$$\text{Prior odds} \times \text{Bayes factor.}$$

Hence, the Bayes Factor, sometimes called the weight of evidence of two hypotheses, is a comparison ratio of how well two hypotheses predict the actual empirical data. Furthermore, we can interpret the Bayes factor as the ratio of credibility of two hypotheses, not as a probability itself. Unlike the p-value, the Bayes factor requires two hypotheses and is contingent on the probability of the observed data alone, not including unobserved "long run" results that are part of the calculation of the p-value. The formula for the Bayes factor allows us to establish the relationship between a minimum Bayes factor required for detecting significance and p-values (see Table A–5 based on Goodman, 1999).

For instance, when an observed value of a sample results in $z = 1.96$ (p-value $= 0.05$), the minimum Bayes factor is 0.15, that is, three times as large as 0.05. This means that the credibility of the null hypothesis is 15% while the credibility of the research hypothesis is 85%. This indicates that the strength

Table A–5. Comparison Between p-Values and the Bayesian Factor and the Evidential Effects on the Null Hypothesis.

Two-Tailed p-Value	Minimum Bayes Factor	Strength of Evidence (Bayesian Conclusion)
0.10 (Z = 1.645)	0.26 (1/3.8)	Weak
0.05 (Z = 1.96)	0.15 (1/6.8)	Weak to Moderate
0.03 (Z = 2.17)	0.095 (1/11)	Moderate
0.01 (Z = 2.58)	0.036 (1/28)	Moderate to Strong
0.001 (Z = 3.28)	0.005 (1/216)	Strong to Very Strong
Less than 0.001	Less than 0.005	Very Strong

of evidence against the null hypothesis is not quite as significant as "$p = 0.05$" actually suggests. Rather, much weaker evidence is derived. The main goal of statistical inference is to quantify uncertainty about unknown facts.

Unlike the p-value approach, the Bayes Factor provides both a framework for quantifying uncertainty of two hypotheses and a method for revising such uncertainty in the light of acquired empirical evidence.

Clinical Applications in the Behavioral and Health Sciences: Description, Graph, and Statistical Analysis

Applications of single subject designs are widespread across diverse areas of clinical practice and research. SSD applications can be found, for example, in clinical studies relating to interventions in stroke, aphasia/speech-motor disorders, hearing loss, autism, attention deficit and hyperactivity disorder, and various avenues of occupational therapy, clinical and rehabilitation psychology, and sports psychology.

In this section of the book, five areas of clinical research/practice are given attention, most of which are also directly concerned with the broader field of communication disorders. It has already been emphasized in the preface that the scope of topics in the behavioral sciences where SSDs can be applied goes well beyond these five areas. Discussion within a handbook requires that this focus be limited to a small set of representative examples.

1. Treatment of anomia in aphasia
2. Treatment of dysarthria
3. General clinical and rehabilitation psychology
4. Assessment of speech and hearing following cochlear implants
5. Training interventions for children with autism

Another factor that influenced the choice of examples has to do with the extent of actual application of specific SSDs (A-B, A-B-A, etc) across the clinical spectrum. Although many areas of communication disorders and psychology utilize SSDs, a good number of sound studies where specific SSDs can be seen applied, does not occur evenly across the clinical spectrum. The five example areas discussed in this section provide a sufficient number of SSD studies from which hypothetical examples can be drawn for the purpose of illustrating SSD analysis.

The format for this section is as follows: A brief description of the clinical area is presented. One or two types of treatment interventions commonly made by communication disorders specialists are described. A few clinical studies are detailed in which SSDs have been used to examine treatment efficacy. A key purpose of this discussion is to bring forth the utility and necessity of SSDs in these clinical situations. Based on the studies described, two hypothetical examples of SSD clinical studies are formulated. The data from these hypothetical examples are tabulated and graphically presented. The data are then analyzed and interpreted with descriptive, inferential and probabilistic methods.

The hypothetical examples are formulated to serve the statistical analysis that follows each set of examples. The examples do not include a critique of the research design (the reader is referred to Part 1 of the book where limitations common to SSDs in general are laid out). To facilitate the statistical analysis, all numerical data are presented in whole numbers.

SECTION A

Single Subject Designs in the Treatment of Anomia in Aphasia

Overview

Single subject research designs are widely used in studies of treatment interventions in aphasia. Many variations can be introduced to some common treatment options aimed at addressing the numerous cognitive manifestations in aphasia. This provides an opportunity in applying single subject designs in aphasia research. One initiative, for example, has to do with further characterizing the manifestations of aphasia especially when they do not match the diagnostic criteria for major types (Young, 2003). The unique aspects of the cognitive profiles among aphasia patients often pose a challenge in describing the disorder and determining optimal treatment methods for each manifestation. Single subject designs for evaluating the efficacy of cognitive treatment of aphasia have been of particular interest (see Kearns, 2000). With particular sets of cognitive impairments in aphasia, comes the need to develop or determine the methods of treatment most suited to the particular impairments (Linebaugh, Shisler, & Lehner, 2005).

Single subject designs prove ideal when dealing with one or a few aphasia patients. They may have a unique set of impairments and the effectiveness of their customized treatment protocols may need to be gauged. The general fostering of evidence-based practice in the treatment of aphasia has also prompted the use of single subject designs (Fucetola, Tucker, Blank, & Corbetta, 2005).

Anomia refers to naming deficits and word-retrieval problems. It is a very common feature of aphasia and is strongly manifested in almost all the syndromes of aphasia (see Caplan, 2003). The patient often shows deficits in naming common objects, symbols, body parts, and colors. In aphasia therapy, much attention is given to the cognitive treatment of anomia. A clinician implementing such treatment may typically need to address questions such as: What kinds of cues work best with a patient with anomia or a certain kind of anomia? What is the optimal rate of presentation (timing) when presenting to the patient either stimuli to test word finding or the cues to aid word finding? What levels of word complexity are best given to a patient?

In this section, we use clinical examples of the treatment of anomia to illustrate the application of single subject designs.

Examples of Studies of the Treatment of Anomia Where Single Subject Designs Have Been Employed

Studies have targeted the treatment of anomia in a variety of ways. Word cuing and phonemic cuing are strategies often used in assisting patients with anomia. Giving a patient a cue about a word can help the patient retrieve the word. Different types of cues and different formats for applying cues make for a range of cuing paradigms, the efficacy of which need to be validated. Freed, Celery, and Marshall (2004) compared the effectiveness of a form of personalized cuing involving novel visual stimuli to phonemic cuing. The research question had to do with the effectiveness of each cue type as measured through the aphasic patients' long-term naming performance. An alternating treatments design (each of the two cuing conditions) was applied on each of three subjects. For each treatment condition, there was a training session (learning the names of common objects) followed by testing sessions at 1 week, 1 month, 2 months, and 3 months. Personalized cuing yielded significantly higher naming performance at 3 months post-training. Wambaugh, Cameron, Kalinyak-Fliszar, et al. (2004) also compared two cuing treatments, phonemic and semantic, but were interested specifically in the potential of the treatments in aiding patients' recall of action words. Multiple baseline and alternating designs were applied on five subjects. The results were mixed, suggesting a possible role for each treatment with different subjects.

Word recall in aphasic patients can also be influenced by the interval pattern or interstimulus interval used in presentation of stimuli (Fridriksson, Holland, & Beeson, 2005). The effects of two types of interval patterns during testing, fixed-spaced and randomized-interval space, were compared by Morrow and Fridriksson (2006) in treating anomia. An alternating treatments design was applied. Three subjects received two alternating treatments (fixed-spaced and randomized-interval) per week. Measured over numerous sessions, both treatments showed success in promoting word recall. No statistically significant difference was found between the two treatment effects.

Kiran and Thompson (2003) examined naming performance in four subjects when they were trained with items presented along successive levels of semantic complexity. For each of two semantic categories, birds and vegetables, items that were typical, intermediate and atypical of the semantic category, were presented, each in a different probe set. Each subject therefore received six probe sets. The sequence for each probe set was, baseline assessment, treatment (naming probes), and follow-up probes at 6 and 10 weeks. Results indicated that subjects were able to generalize their training on atypical semantic categories to the intermediate and typical categories but were not able to generalize from typical categories to the other categories.

In the examples above, single subject designs enabled the researchers to train a few aphasic or anomic individuals in a highly personalized manner. Subjects were trained on very specialized tasks, utilizing complex cuing protocols, involving lengthy and extensive treatment exposure. Follow-up was made over periods up to a few months. The intensity and complexity of the training, its time-consuming nature, the multiple follow-up probes, and communication demands required when working with the subject group in question, make it far less feasible for this kind of research to be conducted expediently on large subject groups.

Examples of Data Sets (two hypothetical cases)

We consider two hypothetical examples of single subject studies addressing the treatment of anomia. In both examples, a single baseline, alternating treatments design is applied.

Example 1

A subject presents with anomia. The clinician conducts a general assessment and infers that the subject's word-finding ability is easily influenced by the interval at which brief statements about the meaning or definition of words are presented. The clinician speculates that if the interval is too short, the patient is not given enough time to consolidate and clear each word or word search before moving on to the next. The clinician now wishes to clarify this effect and begins by comparing two interval conditions. The subject is first given 10 baseline probes. In these probes, sets of word definitions are presented to the subject at random intervals ranging from 1 to 30 seconds following the presentation of the preceding trial. The subject is then given two learning treatments: (a) sets of word definitions presented at uniform, fixed intervals, and (b) a series presented at contingent intervals. In the fixed-intervals treatment, the interstimulus time remains the same (6 seconds) irrespective of whether the subject produces the correct or incorrect response. In the contingent-interval treatment, the interstimulus time is shortened after each correct

response and lengthened after each incorrect response. The two treatment interventions are given in a weekly alternating design over 16 weeks. Each treatment is therefore given 8 times. Each baseline and treatment trial is scored on a 10-point scale. The subject's baseline scores range around the 50% mark. Scores in the contingent-interval condition are found to be similar to the baseline scores. Scores in the fixed interval condition are found to be generally higher than scores in the contingent interval condition. Table A–1 and Figure A–1 illustrate the data.

The clinician applied a simple alternating treatment design to get a quick gauge of the subject's preference for one or the other patterns of stimulus intervals. With this data, the clinician can now design longer course of treatment for the patient and apply a fixed-interval pattern in stimulus presentation. Go to Statistical Analysis for Example 1.

Example 2

A subject presents with moderate anomia. The clinician perceives that the subject's word-finding difficulties are not generalized but appear to be more pronounced with some semantic categories. The clinician chooses to compare the subject's performance in word-finding tasks across different semantic categories of words. One of the clinician's experiments examines the subject's naming accuracy between the semantic categories of (a) kitchenware and (b) types of clothing. Picture-naming tests are used. The study begins with 10 sessions of baseline testing using typical items from many semantic categories. Ten intervention sessions are then given in which word examples from each of the two semantic categories of interest are presented. A weekly alternating design is used—there are five intervention sessions for each semantic category. Follow-up probes are

Table A–1. Subject's word-naming scores in the baseline condition and the fixed- and contingent-interval conditions of presentation of word meanings.

(a)

Number of Contact Words in 10 Random Interval Patterns	5	4	6	5	7	4	3	7	5	4
Trials	1	2	3	4	5	6	7	8	9	10
	Baseline									

(b)

The two intervention conditions alternated weekly over 16 weeks.

Number of Correct Words in Fixed Interval Condition	6	8	7	8	8	7	8	8
Number of Correct Words in Contingent Interval Condition	5	6	6	7	5	4	4	6
	11	12	13	14	15	16	17	18
	Treatment							

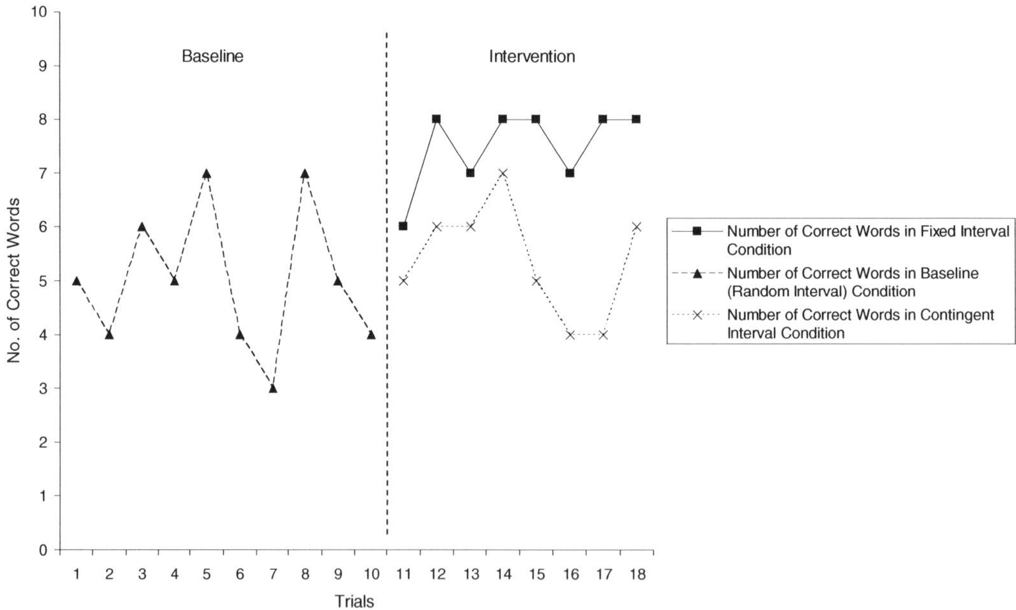

Figure A–1. Graphical representation of subject's word naming scores in the baseline condition and the fixed- and contingent-interval conditions of presentation of word meanings.

given at 12 and 14 weeks. All trials are scored on a 10-point scale. Baseline scores are found to be variable around the 40% mark. Scores for the words in the category of kitchen items are found to be in the 50% mark. Scores for the category of clothing are found to be consistently greater, around the 70% mark. Table A–2 and Figure A–2 illustrate the data. Go to Statistical Analysis for Example 2.

The single subject design revealed a difference in performance between the two conditions. The clinician can now apply this framework to investigate the subject's word-finding patterns across other semantic categories.

Table A–2. Subject's word-naming scores for words from many semantic categories (baseline condition) and words from the semantic categories of clothing and kitchen items.

(a)

Number of Correct Words Across Many Semantic Categories	5	4	4	6	3	4	3	5	4	5
Trials	1	2	3	4	5	6	7	8	9	10
	Baseline									

(b)

The two intervention conditions alternated weekly over 16 weeks.

Number of Correct Words for Clothing Items	7	8	8	6	7	8	7	7	6	7
Number of Correct Words for Kitchenware Items	5	7	6	4	4	6	5	7	4	5
	11	12	13	14	15	16	17	18	19	20
	Treatment									

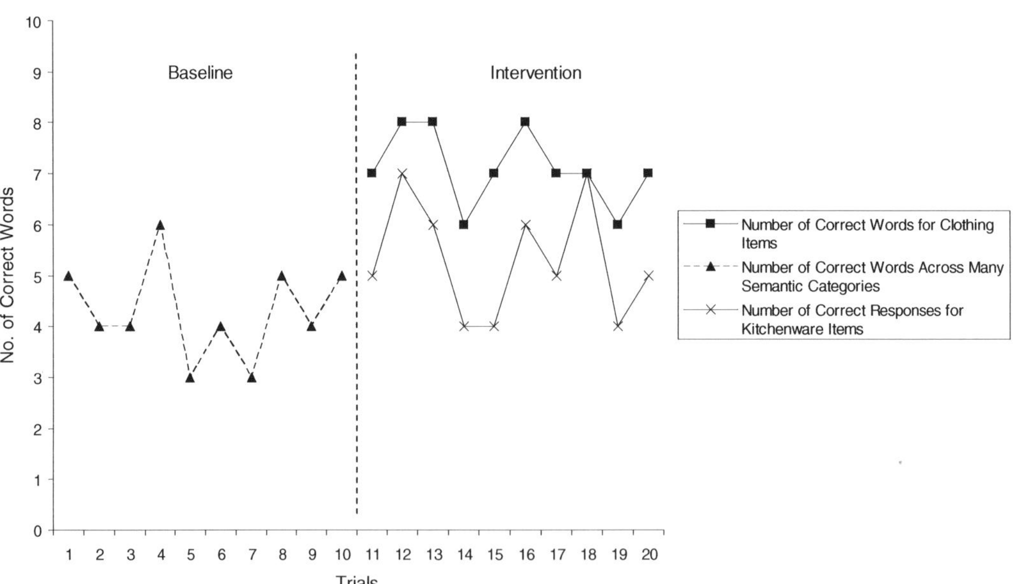

Figure A–2. Graphical representation of subject's word naming scores in the baseline condition and the two treatment conditions.

STATISTICAL ANALYSIS FOR EXAMPLE 1

Data from Table A–1: Subject's word-naming scores (Number of correct words in Fixed Interval Conditions)—AB Design.

A_1 = Baseline 1, B_1 = Intervention 1

Using the statistical software packages, like SPSS, SAS, MINITAB 14, and so on, we can perform several analyses as follows.

1. Descriptive Statistics

A_1: MEAN = 5.00, MEDIAN = 5, SD = 1.333, $n = 10$

B_1: MEAN = 7.50, MEDIAN = 8, SD = 0.755, $n = 8$

Correlation Coefficients: r (A_1 and B_1) = 0.206

μ (A_1 and B_1) = 6.11

2. Analysis of Variance

a. For the two phases (A_1 and B_1)

Sources	SS	df	MS = SS/df	F	p	Significance*
Between	27.778	1	27.778	22.222	<0.01	Highly significant
Within	20	16	1.25			

*We use the terms "Highly significant" when $p <.01$, "significant" when $.01 \leq p <.05$, and "Not significant" when $p \geq .05$. In the author's view, the level of significance (p value) reported cannot necessarily be equated with the magnitude of the treatment effect.

3. Autocorrelation Coefficients-Product-Moment lag-1

A_1: $r = -0.323, p = 0.39508$

B_1: $r = -0.496, p = 0.25744$

4. Mann-Whitney U Test

a. For the first two phases (A_1 and B_1)

U = 4.5, $Z = 3.15, p <0.01$ (Highly significant)

5. t-test

a. For the first two phases (A_1 and B_1)

$t(16) = 4.714, p = 0.000$ (Highly significant)

6. Time Series Analysis

Phases	C	$Z = C/SE$	p-value	Significance
A_1	−0.281	−0.989	0.838	Not significant
B_1	0.000	0.000	0.500	Not significant
A_1 and B_1	0.445	2.000	0.022	Significant

Where SE = SQR $[(n-2)/(n+1)(n-1)]$, C = $1-[\Sigma(X_i-X_{i+1})^2/2\Sigma(X-\mu)^2]$, and

Z = C/SE

7. Bayesian Analysis

Hypothesis: H_o: No Effect, H_a: An Effect Exists

a. For the first two phases (A_1 and B_1)

Data	(X_i-X_{i+1})	$(X_i-X_{i+1})^2$	$(X-\mu)$	$(X-\mu)^2$	Phases
5	1	1	−1.11	1.2321	A_1
4	−2	4	−2.11	4.4521	
6	1	1	−0.11	0.0121	
5	−2	4	−1.11	1.2321	
7	3	9	0.89	0.7921	
4	1	1	−2.11	4.4521	
3	−4	16	−3.11	9.6721	
7	2	4	0.89	0.7921	
5	1	1	−1.11	1.2321	
4	−2	4	−2.11	4.4521	
6	−2	4	−0.11	0.0121	B_1
8	1	1	1.89	3.5721	
7	−1	1	0.89	0.7921	
8	0	0	1.89	3.5721	
8	1	1	1.89	3.5721	
7	−1	1	0.89	0.7921	
8	0	0	1.89	3.5721	
8	—	—	1.89	3.5721	
SUM (Σ)		53		47.7778	

Therefore, we can obtain the values of C, SD, and Z (by the formulas shown under Time-Series Analysis) as follows.

$n = 18$, SE = 0.2226, $C = 0.4453$, and $Z = 2.000$ ($p = 0.022$ is also called "Likelihood").

Keep repeating this process, we will eventually be able to calculate Likelihood, Bayes Factor (the ratio of likelihoods), and posterior probability of each consecutive phases (See Questions 34 and 36 in Part I for further details.). The following table shows a summary of the results of each phase.

Phases	Hypothesis	Prior Probability	Likelihood	Bayes Factor (λ)	Prior $\times$ Likelihood	Posterior Probability	
A_1B_1	H_o	0.5	0.022	0.0225	0.011	0.022	Moderate to Strong Treatment Effect*
	H_a	0.5	0.978		0.489	0.978	

*The strength of evidence during the first two phases showed that the first treatment is Moderate to Strong.

8. Celeration Line

Figure A–3 (first two phases A_1B_1 in fixed interval conditions) is the celeration line of this AB Design. (For further details, readers should review Question 12 in Part I.)

9. χ^2 Analysis

Phases	Below (Undesired)*	Above (Desired)**
A_1	4	6
B_1	8	0

* and **: Below or Above the Celeration Line. See Part I for further details.

χ^2 ($n = 18$) = 7.2, p <0.01 (Highly significant)

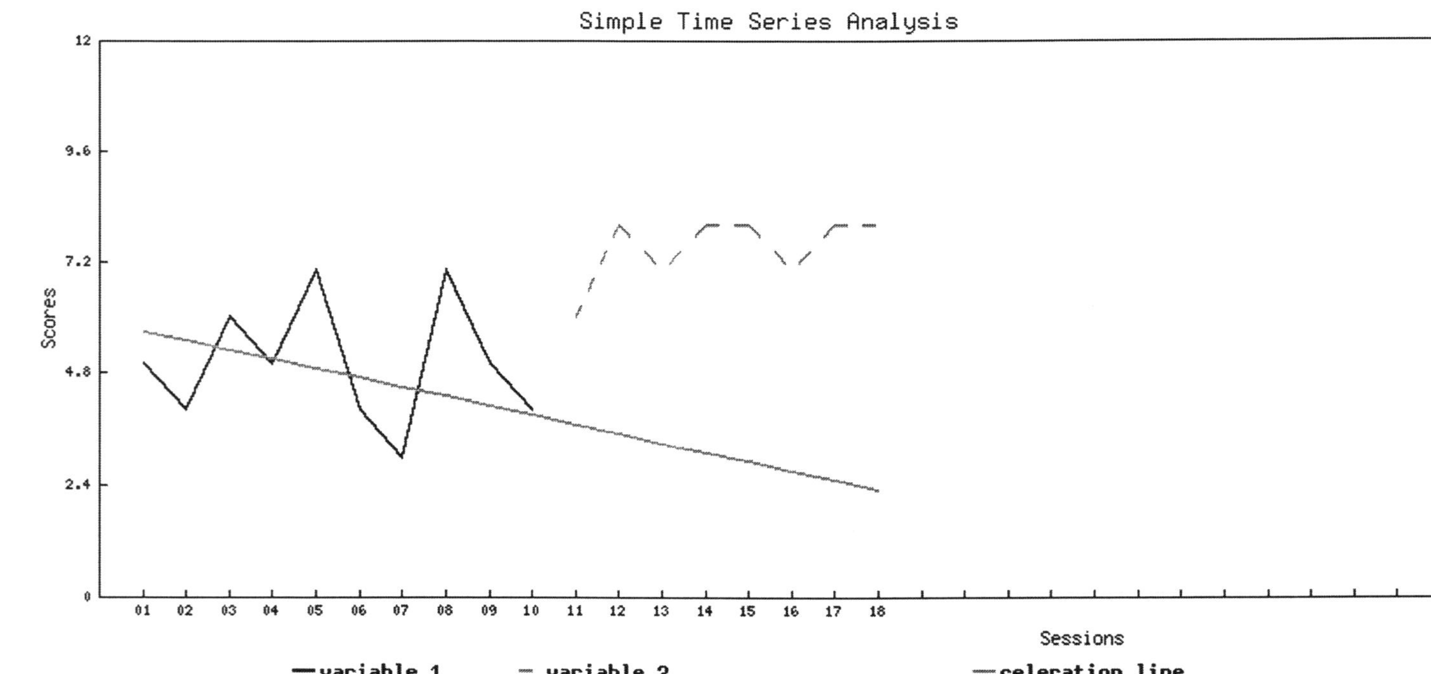

Figure A–3. First two phases A_1B_1 in fixed interval conditions (A_1 = Variable 1, B_1 = Variable 2).

STATISTICAL ANALYSIS FOR EXAMPLE 1

Data from Table A–1. Subject's word-naming scores (Number of correct words in Contingent Interval Conditions)—AB Design.

A_1 = Baseline 1, B_1 = Intervention 1

Using the statistical software packages, like SPSS, SAS, MINITAB 14, and so on, we can perform several analyses as follows.

1. Descriptive Statistics

A_1: MEAN = 5.00, MEDIAN = 5, SD = 1.333, $n = 10$

B_1: MEAN = 5.37, MEDIAN = 5.50, SD = 1.060, $n = 8$

Correlation Coefficients: r (A_1 and B_1) = 0.339

μ (A_1 and B_1) = 5.167

2. Analysis of Variance

a. For the two phases (A_1 and B_1)

Sources	SS	df	MS = SS/df	F	p	Significance
Between	0.625	1	0.625	0.419	0.5267	Not significant
Within	23.875	16	1.492			

3. Autocorrelation Coefficients-Product-Moment lag-1

A_1: $r = -0.323, p = 0.39508$

B_1: $r = -0.283, p = 0.53847$

4. Mann-Whitney U Test

a. For the first two phases (A_1 and B_1)

U = 32.5, $Z = 0.66, p > 0.05$ (Not significant)

5. t-test

a. For the first two phases (A_1 and B_1)

$t(16) = 0.647, p = 0.526$ (Not significant)

6. Time Series Analysis

Phases	C	$Z = C/SE$	p-value	Significance
A_1	−0.281	−0.989	0.838	Not significant
B_1	0.301	0.977	0.164	Not significant
A_1 and B_1	−0.081	−0.366	0.643	Not significant

Where $SE = SQR[(n-2)/(n+1)(n-1)]$, $C = 1-[\Sigma(X_i-X_{i+1})^2/2\Sigma(X-\mu)^2]$, and $Z = C/SE$

7. Bayesian Analysis

Hypothesis: H_o: No Effect, H_a: An Effect Exists

a. For the first two phases (A_1 and B_1)

Data	(X_i-X_{i+1})	$(X_i-X_{i+1})^2$	$(X-\mu)$	$(X-\mu)^2$	Phases
5	1	1	−0.167	0.027889	A_1
4	−2	4	−1.167	1.362	
6	1	1	0.833	0.6939	
5	−2	4	−0.167	0.027889	
7	3	9	1.833	3.36	
4	1	1	−1.167	1.362	
3	−4	16	−2.167	4.70	
7	2	4	1.833	3.36	
5	1	1	−0.167	0.027889	
4	−2	4	−1.167	1.362	
5	−1	1	−0.167	0.027889	B_1
6	0	0	0.833	0.6939	
6	−1	1	0.833	0.6939	
7	2	4	1.833	3.36	
5	1	1	−0.167	0.027889	
4	0	0	−1.167	1.362	
4	−2	4	−1.167	1.362	
6	—	—	0.833	0.6939	
SUM (Σ)		53		24.505	

Therefore, we can obtain the values of C, SD, and Z (by the formulas shown under Time-Series Analysis) as follows.

$n = 18$, SE $= 0.2226$, $C = -0.0818$, and $Z = -0.3675$ ($p = 0.643$ is also called "Likelihood").

Keep repeating this process, we will eventually be able to calculate Likelihood, Bayes factor (the ratio of likelihoods), and posterior probability of each consecutive phases (See Questions 34 and 36 in Part I for further details).

The following table shows a summary of the results of each phase.

Phases	Hypothesis	Prior Probability	Likelihood	Bayes Factor (λ)	Prior × Likelihood	Posterior Probability	
A_1B_1	H_o	0.5	0.643	1.80	0.3215	0.643	Very Weak Treatment Effect*
	H_a	0.5	0.357		0.1785	0.357	

*The strength of evidence during the first two phases showed that the first treatment is Very Weak.

8. Celeration Line

Figure A–4 (First two phases A_1B_1 in contingent interval conditions) is the celeration line of this AB Design. (For further details, readers should review Question 12 in Part I.)

Insert Figure A–4 First two phases A_1B_1

9. χ^2 Analysis

Phases	Below (Undesired)*	Above (Desired)**
A_1	4	6
B_1	8	0

* and **: Below or Above the Celeration Line. See Part I for further details.

χ^2 ($n = 18$) $= 7.2$, $p < 0.01$ (Highly significant)

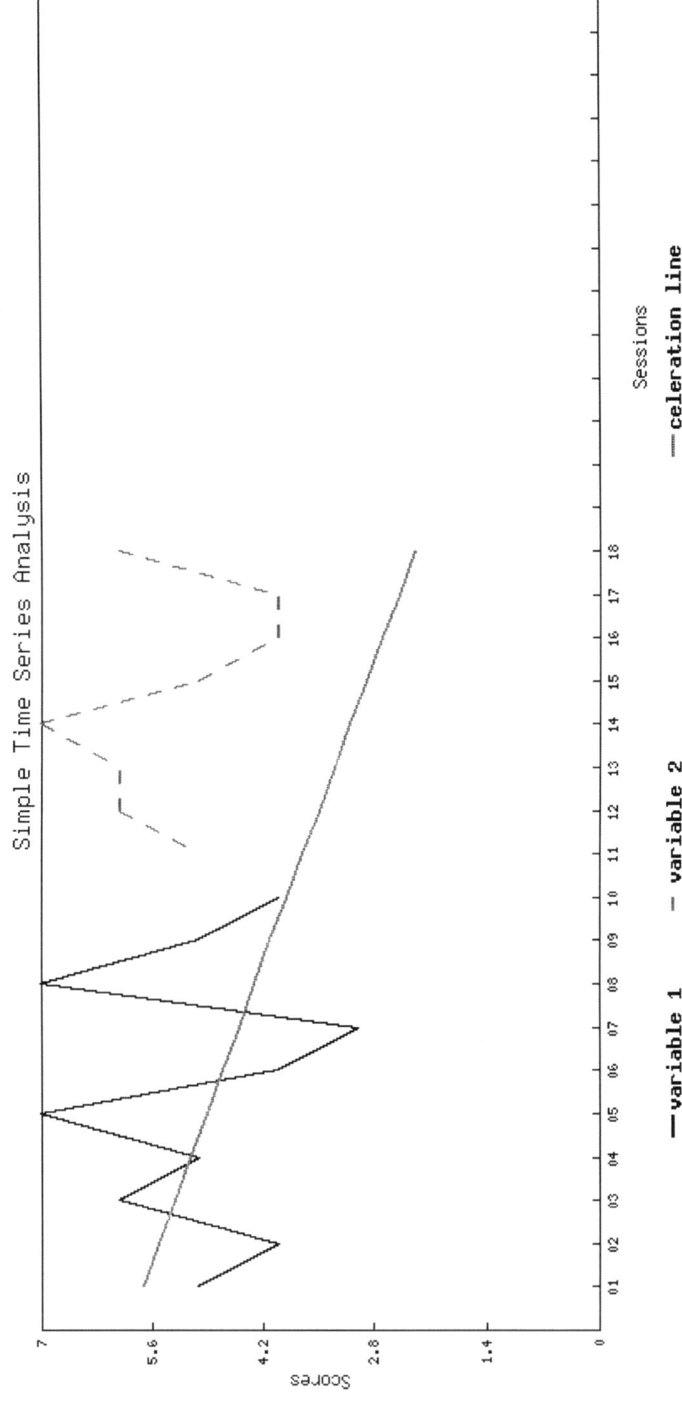

Figure A–4. First two phases A_1B_1 in contingent interval conditions (A_1 = Variable 1, B_1 = Variable 2).

STATISTICAL ANALYSIS FOR EXAMPLE 2

Data from Table A–2: Subject's word-naming scores for (a) words from many semantic categories (baseline condition) and (b) words from the semantic categories of clothing and kitchen items—AB Design.

A_1 = Baseline 1, B_1 = Intervention 1

Using the statistical software packages, like SPSS, SAS, MINITAB 14, and so on, we can perform several analyses as follows.

Clothing Items

1. **Descriptive Statistics**

    A_1: MEAN = 4.30, MEDIAN = 4, SD = 0.948, n =10

    B_1: MEAN = 7.10, MEDIAN = 7, SD = 0.737, n = 10

    Correlation Coefficients: r (A_1 and B_1) = −0.365

    μ (A_1 and B_1) = 5.70

2. **Analysis of Variance**

    a. For the two phases (A_1 and B_1)

Sources	SS	df	MS = SS/df	F	p	Significance
Between	39.2	1	39.2	54.277	<0.0001	Highly significant
Within	13.0	18	0.722			

3. **Autocorrelation Coefficients-Product-Moment lag-1**

    A_1: r = −0.455, p = 0.21747

    B_1: r = −0.022, p = 0.95372

4. **Mann-Whitney U Test**

    For the first two phases (A_1 and B_1)

    U = 1.0, Z = 3.70, p <0.01 (Highly significant)

5. **t-test**

    For the first two phases (A_1 and B_1)

    t(18) = 7.367, p = 0.000 (Highly significant)

6. Time Series Analysis

Phases	C	$Z = C/SE$	p-value	Significance
A_1	−0.358	−1.259	0.895	Not significant
B_1	−0.020	−0.071	0.528	Not significant
A_1 and B_1	0.655	3.084	0.001	Highly significant

Where $SE = SQR\ [(n−2)/(n+1)(n−1)]$, $C = 1−[\Sigma(X_i−X_{i+1})^2/2\Sigma(X−\mu)^2]$, and $Z = C/SE$

7. Bayesian Analysis

Hypothesis: H_o: No Effect, H_a: An Effect Exists

a. For the first two phases (A_1 and B_1)

Data	$(X_i−X_{i+1})$	$(X_i−X_{i+1})^2$	$(X−\mu)$	$(X−\mu)^2$	Phases
5	1	1	−0.7	0.49	A_1
4	0	0	−1.7	2.89	
4	−2	4	−1.7	2.8	
6	3	9	0.3	0.09	
3	−1	1	−2.7	7.29	
4	1	1	−1.7	2.89	
3	−2	4	−2.7	7.29	
5	1	1	−0.7	0.49	
4	−1	1	−1.7	2.89	
5	−2	4	−0.7	0.49	
7	−1	1	1.3	1.69	B_1
8	0	0	2.3	5.29	
8	2	4	2.3	5.29	
6	−1	1	0.3	0.09	
7	−1	1	1.3	1.69	
8	1	1	2.3	5.29	
7	0	0	1.3	1.69	
7	1	1	1.3	1.69	
6	−1	1	0.3	0.09	
7	—	—	1.3	1.69	
Sum (Σ)		36		52.20	

Therefore, we can obtain the values of C, SD, and Z (by the formulas shown under Time-Series Analysis) as follows:

$n = 20$, SE $= 0.21240$, $C = 0.65517$, and $Z = 3.08$ ($p = 0.001$ is also called "Likelihood").

Keep repeating this process, we will eventually be able to calculate Likelihood, Bayes Factor (the ratio of likelihoods), and posterior probability of each consecutive phases (See Questions 34 and 36 in Part I for further details).

The following table shows a summary of the results of each phase.

Phases	Hypothesis	Prior Probability	Likelihood	Bayes Factor (λ)	Prior × Likelihood	Posterior Probability	
A_1B_1	H_o	0.5	0.001	0.001	0.0005	0.001	Strong to Very Strong Treatment Effect*
	H_a	0.5	0.999		0.4995	0.999	

*The strength of evidence during the first two phases showed that the first treatment is Strong to Very Strong.

8. Celeration Line

Figure A–5 (first two phases A_1B_1 of clothing items shown below) is the celeration line of this AB Design.(For further details, readers should review Question 12 in Part I)

9. χ^2 Analysis

Phases	Below (Undesired)*	Above (Desired)**
A_1	4	6
B_1	10	0

* and **: Below or Above the Celeration Line. See Part I for further details.

χ^2 ($n = 20$) = 8.571, $p <0.01$ (Highly significant)

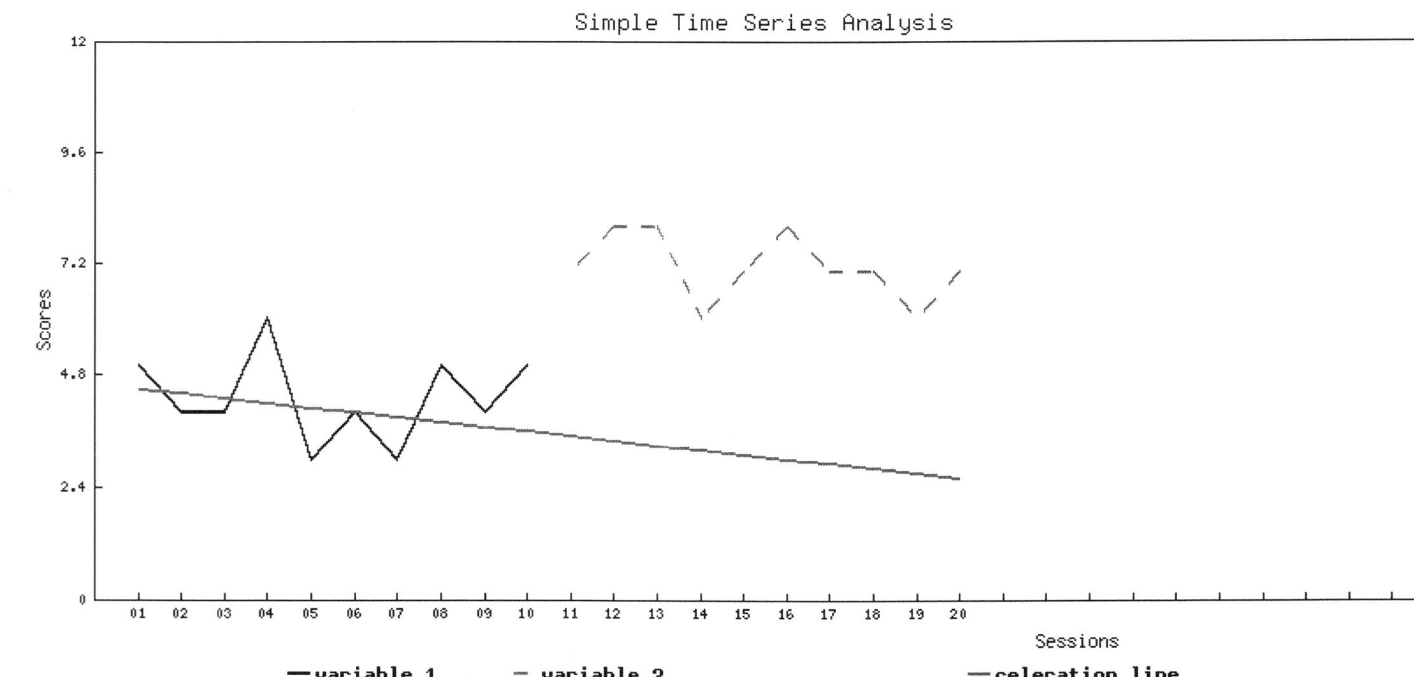

Figure A–5. First two phases A_1B_1 of clothing items (A_1 = Variable 1, B_1 = Variable 2).

Kitchenware Items

1. Descriptive Statistics

A_1: MEAN = 4.30, MEDIAN = 4, SD = 0.948, n = 10

B_1: MEAN = 5.30, MEDIAN = 5, SD = 1.159, n = 10

Correlation Coefficients: r (A_1 and B_1) = 0.010

μ (A_1 and B_1) = 4.80

2. Analysis of Variance

a. For the two phases (A_1 and B_1)

Sources	SS	df	MS = SS/df	F	p	Significance
Between	5.0	1	5.0	4.455	0.049	Significant
Within	20.2	18	1.122			

3. Autocorrelation Coefficients-Product-Moment lag-1

A_1: r = -0.455, p = 0.21747

B_1: r = -0.166, p = 0.66823

4. Mann-Whitney U Test

For the first two phases (A_1 and B_1)

U = 26.5, Z = 1.77, p >0.05 (Not significant)

5. t-test

For the first two phases (A_1 and B_1)

t(18) = 2.110, p = 0.049 (Significant)

6. Time Series Analysis

Phases	C	Z = C/SE	p-value	Significance
A_1	−0.358	−1.259	0.895	Not significant
B_1	−0.157	−0.552	0.709	Not significant
A_1 and B_1	0.007	0.037	0.485	Not significant

Where SE = SQR$[(n-2)/(n+1)(n-1)]$, $C = 1-[\Sigma(X_i-X_{i+1})^2/2\Sigma(X-\mu)^2]$, and Z = C/SE

7. Bayesian Analysis

Hypothesis: H_o: No Effect, H_a: An Effect Exists

a. For the first two phases (A_1 and B_1)

Data	(X_i-X_{i+1})	$(X_i-X_{i+1})^2$	$(X-\mu)$	$(X-\mu)^2$	Phases
5	1	1	0.2	0.04	A_1
4	0	0	−0.8	0.64	
4	−2	4	−0.8	0.64	
6	3	9	1.2	1.44	
3	−1	1	−1.8	3.24	
4	1	1	−0.8	0.64	
3	−2	4	−1.8	3.24	
5	1	1	0.2	0.04	
4	−1	1	−0.8	0.64	
5	0	0	0.2	0.04	
5	−2	4	0.2	0.04	B_1
7	1	1	2.2	4.84	
6	2	4	1.2	1.44	
4	0	0	−0.8	0.64	
4	−2	4	−0.8	0.64	
6	1	1	1.2	1.44	
5	−2	4	0.2	0.04	
7	3	9	2.2	4.84	
4	−1	1	−0.8	0.64	
5	—	—	0.2	0.04	
Sum (Σ)		50		25.20	

Therefore, we can obtain the values of C, SD, and Z (by the formulas shown under Time-Series Analysis) as follows.

$N = 20$, SE $= 0.21240$, $C = 0.0079365$, and $Z = 0.03737$ ($p = 0.485$ is also called "Likelihood").

Keep repeating this process, we will eventually be able to calculate Likelihood, Bayes Factor (the ratio of likelihoods), and posterior probability of each consecutive phases (See Questions 34 and 36 in Part I for further details).

The following table shows a summary of the results of each phase.

Phases	Hypothesis	Prior Probability	Likelihood	Bayes Factor (λ)	Prior × Likelihood	Posterior Probability	
A_1B_1	H_o	0.5	0.485	0.9417	0.2425	0.485	Very Weak Treatment Effect*
	H_a	0.5	0.515		0.2575	0.515	

*The strength of evidence during the first two phases showed that the first treatment is Very Weak.

8. Celeration Line

Figure A–6 (first two phases A_1B_1 of kitchenware items shown below) is the celeration line of this AB Design. (For further details, readers should review Question 12 in Part I.)

9. χ^{-2} Analysis

Phases	Below (Undesired)*	Above (Desired)**
A_1	4	6
B_1	10	0

* and **: Below or above the Celeration Line. See Part I for further details.

χ^{-2} ($n = 20$) = 8.571, p <0.01 (Highly significant)

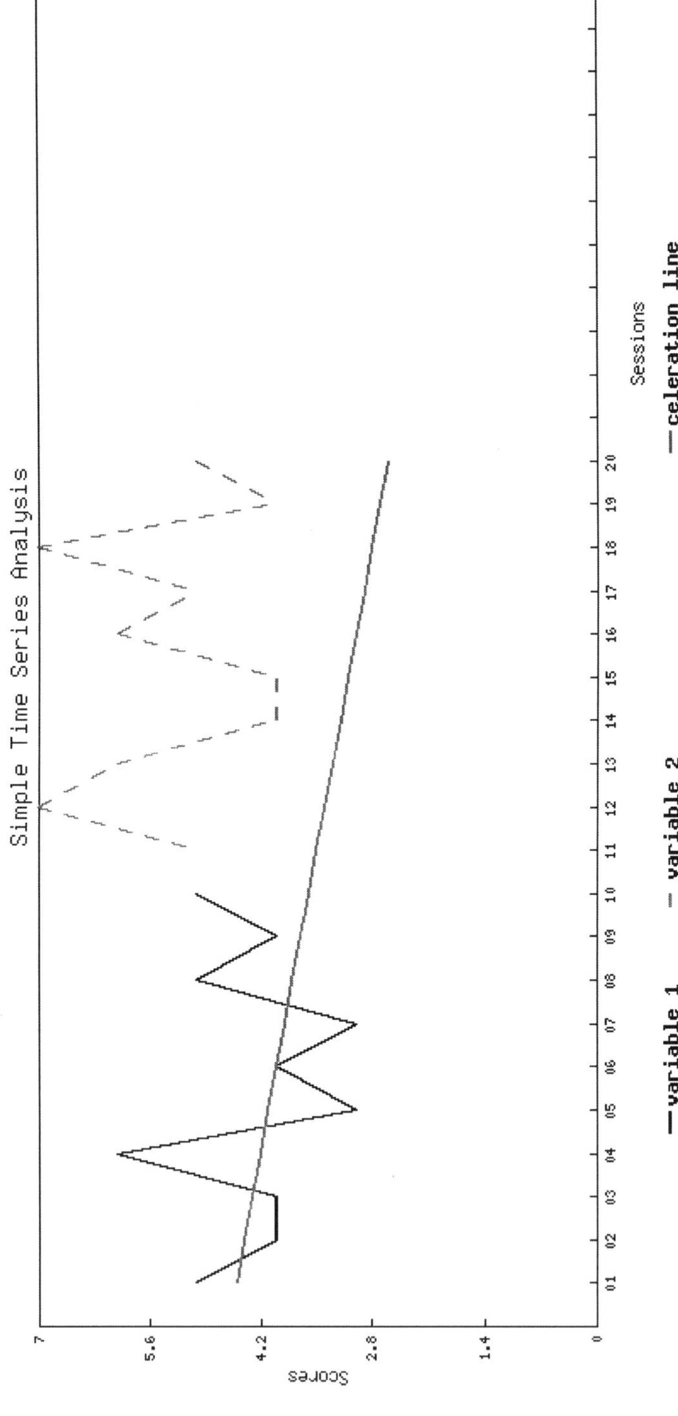

Figure A–6. First two phases A_1B_1 of kitchenware items (A_1 = Variable 1, B_1 = Variable 2).

54

SECTION B

Single Subject Designs in the Treatment of Dysarthria

Overview

Clinicians in communication disorders face a range of clinical syndromes where dysarthria features prominently. Dysarthria is a neurologic-motor condition in which a variety of speech motor systems may be affected. It is characterized by slowness, weakness, and incoordination of the speech musculature that manifest in imprecise speech, poor rate or pitch of speech, or even severely reduced speech (Kaye, 2000). Imprecise respiratory, phonatory, and articulatory aspects of speech are also commonly present. Dysarthric speech patterns can vary widely. The range of speech symptoms and etiology in patients with dysarthia are therefore more accurately characterized as a group of disorders, "the dysarthrias" (Simpson, Till, & Goff, 1988; Yorkston, 1996). Dysarthria may result from congenital conditions such as cerebral palsy, or acquired conditions such as stroke, traumatic brain injury, and Parkinson's disease.

The varied patterns of dysarthria as well as the chronic nature of the condition call for a special role of speech-language clinicians in diagnosis and treatment. After identifying the type of dysarthria presented by a patient, its severity, and specific symptoms, the clinician has to select or tailor an intervention for speech improvement (see Yorkston, 1996; Yorkston, Beukelman, & Bell, 1988). In doing so, the clinician also faces some specific problems. The efficacy of different forms of interventions for dysarthria has not been well researched (Duffy, 1995) and variations in dysarthric patterns in individuals over the long term are not well understood (Simpson et al., 1988). Focusing on individual cases or applying single subject designs constitutes a way of addressing these shortcomings. The single subject approach is of particular relevance when dealing with dysarthria in that it can accommodate a highly individualized, patient-centered diagnostic profile and treatment plan (Yorkston, 1996). The single case or single subject design can also conveniently accommodate a variety or treatment options and measurement techniques that may have to be applied in the course of a patient's long-term treatment. More recent dysarthria rehabilitation approaches are influenced by neurobiologic views of speech production and gives attention to specific speech production mechanisms

(Murdoch, Pitt, Theodoros, & Ward, 1999). Single subject designs again lend themselves ideally to this approach where a treatment variable isolated in one patient may be quite different from that of another patient and where the efficacy of an intervention may have to be assessed individually.

Examples of Research Studies in Dysarthria Where Single Subject Designs Have Been Employed

The following studies provide examples of the use of single subject designs in the treatment of dysarthria. Havstam, Buchholz, and Hartelius (2003) examined the effectiveness of an augmentative, computer-based speech recognition system on two patients with severe dysarthia secondary to cerebral palsy. Among other functions, the computer system was designed to take samples and store templates of the patient's speech, interpret the patient's speech, and compare the patient's speech production to the stored templates. In this system, the progression of the computerized task was dependent on the computer's recognition of the patients' spoken word. The researchers were interested in finding out if the system could benefit patients with severe dysarthria or anarthria, and if the system could augment an original, more conventional computerized system. Their study involved two subjects. A few baseline measurements were taken. These included (1) a measure of the patients' efficiency in accessing the original computer system, using a text copying/speech recognition task, and (2) a measure of the patient's speech production using a word-sentence repetition task and a picture-naming task. The newer speech recognition computer system was then introduced over 4 to 6 training sessions. This was followed by measurements of system access efficiency and levels of speech recognition. One of the subjects did not complete all phases of the study. The other patient showed a 40% gain on the speech recognition task but no increase in speech production. The study showed that certain modifications to computerized speech recognition systems can aid in increasing speech recognition even in patient with severe dysarthria.

Simpson, Till, and Goff (1988) conducted a study on a single patient with severe dysarthria. The researchers addressed the lack of available data on how speech symptoms can vary over the long term in dysarthric patients. The study involved varied forms of treatment and measurements carried out over a long term (about 3 years) on a single patient. Specific problems relating communication, articulation, respiration for speech, hypernasality, and speech intensity, were addressed in sequence over the course of management, each with a treatment method appropriate to the problem. Following some success in treatment of a problem, the management of the next problem would begin. Treatment of a particular problem could involve many sessions and could extend over many months. None of the treatment methods alone produced any large improvement over the behavior targeted. However, altogether, the small gains from each course of treatment led to marked improvement in the patient's communication and everyday functioning. The study highlighted the effects of periodic interventions over the long term in treating dysarthria, and also the use of particular measurement techniques to gauge small changes over the course of management.

An A-B-A-B design was applied by Murdoch et al. (1999) in assessing the efficacy of two types of feedback methods used to modify speech breathing patterns in dysarthria. The study involved a single subject, a child with persistent dysarthria following traumatic brain injury. The study's central research issue was the comparison of two therapeutic feedback techniques for speech therapy: (1) traditional therapeutic methods that emphasize feedback about the patient's posture, inhalation, general motor performance, and so on (such feedback is generally noncontinuous) and (2) continuous biofeedback, in particular, biofeedback of the patient's rib cage circumference to index the use of the respiratory musculature, as patients with dysarthria secondary to traumatic brain injury are less effective in using their respiratory musculature. The baseline phase A_1 extended over 2 days and involved numerous assessments of the patient's breathing. Speech breathing was found to be severely impaired. The intervention phase B_1 extended over 2 weeks and involved 30 sessions of traditional therapy, using various traditional techniques. Traditional therapy led to a reduction in poor rib cage movements. No other significant improvements were noted. A 10-week long withdrawal phase, A_2, followed. In this phase, assessments of the patient's breathing were made but no therapy was involved. The variables measured did not simply return to baseline levels except for one measure. There was great variability in these measurements. The second intervention phase, B_2, extended over 2 weeks and involved 8 sessions of biofeedback. In this phase, significant physiologic changes were seen on all kinematic (ribcage movement) measures were targeted by the continuous biofeedback. The study neatly demonstrated the effectiveness of visual biofeedback over traditional feedback techniques when applied to a particular case of persistent dysarthria.

It also pointed to the potential of other forms of biofeedback in treating dysarthria by targeting specific speech production mechanisms.

The studies described above illustrate the multitude of symptoms involved in dysarthria, the many ways of assessing and treating the condition, and its variability over the course of treatment. These studies also demonstrate how single subject designs can be used to target particular assessment and treatment variables so as to afford investigations that are feasible and practical. In managing dysarthria, the clinician may often need to manipulate some treatment variables in order to establish a management protocol.

Examples of Data Sets (two hypothetical cases)

We consider two cases, both with A-B-A-B designs where treatment variables and feedback methods are manipulated.

Example 1

A geriatric patient with Parkinson's disease presents with dysarthria. After assessing the patient, the clinician decides to engage the patient in a long-term course of treatment. Because many parts of the treatment will involve presentation of sentences to the patient, the clinician decides to first clarify the type of sentence presentation that yields the best repetition (speech production) from the patient. The patient's slight short-term memory problem is also a factor that the clinician has to consider when deciding on the rate of sentence presentation. One of the clinician's treatment protocols that aims at establishing rate of sentence presentation, contrasts two rate conditions, a phrase-spaced condition and an evenly word-spaced condition. The study begins with the baseline condition (A_1) in which the patient verbally reproduces 10 pairs of sentences read by the clinician. The clinician reads each sentence at a normal speech rate. A general assessment of the patient's sentence production (repetition) is made using a 1 to 10 scale. An average score for each sentence pair is used. Baseline scores are found to be around the halfway mark on the scale. In the first intervention (B_1) carried over 2 days, a second set of 10 pairs of sentences are read to the patient. The procedure is the same as that of (A_1) except that the sentences are presented with a 1.5-second break placed between phrases (for example, in the sentence, "The boy kicked the ball and then ran after it," a 1.5-second interval is placed after "the boy," after "kicked the ball," and after the final phrase). The patient's scores are only slightly above baseline scores. A 2-day withdrawal period (A_2) follows during which the patient reproduces the sentences from the baseline phase (A_1). Performance levels appear to be identical to the baseline levels. The second intervention B_2 then follows over 2 days. The procedure is the same as that of B_1 except that the clinician presents each sentence with 1-second intervals between the words. The sentence set presented is similar but not identical to the set used in B_1. The patient's performance improves to about a 75% level on the scale. Table B–1 and Figure B–1 illustrate the data.

The study reveals that the patient has better success with an evenly spaced word interval in sentence presentation, when contrasted with phrase-spaced sentence presentation. The clinician can design therapeutic tasks accordingly. The results of the study may also point to certain relation-ships between the patients cognitive and dysarthria profiles. Go to Statistical Analysis for Example 1.

Example 2

A teenage patient presents with dysarthria secondary to traumatic brain injury. After assessment, the clinician decides to use a computerized voice-recognition system in the course of treatment. The system works by trying to recognize the words in the patient's spoken sentence; it then attempts to regenerate the sentence produced aloud by the patient. The clinician has had success in using this system for treatment in the past. The clinician also thinks that a more entertaining (video) feedback display could be incorporated into the system to make it more appealing to some pediatric populations, and hence possibly more effective. A treatment protocol is designed first to apply the system without any modifications, and then apply it with the use of computer gamelike animations for feedback. All phases, A_1, B_1, A_2, and B_2, will have 10 scored trials. Ten baseline measures (A_1) are taken in a day using a standard quality of articulation rating scale. The patient repeats the sentence three times after the clinician. The clinician provides therapeutic guidance and instruction between repetitions. Sentence articulation is scored on the third repetition. The clinician uses a 1 to 5 rating scale to assign a score for each trial. Intervention (B_1) follows. The patient produces a set of sentences: The patient's rendering of a sentence is recorded by the computer and the computer attempts to recognize the words. The computer's level of success with word recognition is displayed to the patient as a simple bar graph (on a simple low-middle-high scale). The clinician then provides therapeutic guidance

Table B–1. Patient's scores on Sentence Production in Baseline, First Intervention, Withdrawal, and Second Intervention Phases

Sentence Production Score	4 5 5 6 5 6 3 4 6 7	6 7 7 6 5 4 6 5 5 6	5 4 7 6 6 4 5 4 7 6	8 7 8 6 8 7 9 8 7 7
Trials	1 2 3 4 5 6 7 8 9 10	11 12 13 14 15 16 17 18 19 20	21 22 23 24 25 26 27 28 29 30	31 32 33 34 35 36 37 38 39 40
	Baseline (A$_1$)	Intervention (B$_1$)	Withdrawal (A$_2$)	Intervention (B$_2$)

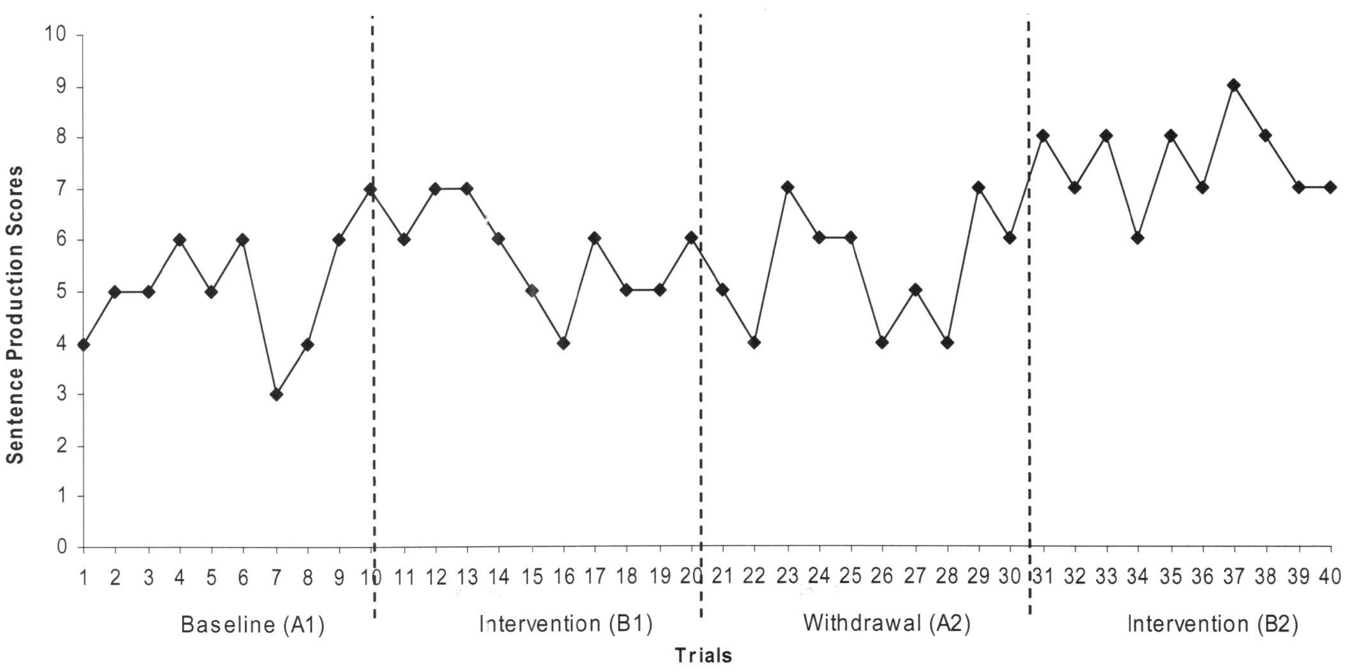

Figure B–1. Graphical illustration of patient's Sentence Production across each phase of the A-B–A-B study.

and instruction. The sequence of sentence production, computer feedback and clinician instruction are repeated for the sentence and, again, rating of the reproduction is made on the third rendering. Average performance exceeds that of the baseline level but the improvement is not remarkable. In the next phase (A_2) the procedure carried out in B_1 is repeated except that computer feedback and clinician input are withdrawn. Average performance slightly exceeds the baseline level. In the last phase (B_2), the procedures used in B_1 are repeated but the plain bar graph computer feedback is accompanied with an animated cartoon sequence and sounds when the bar exceeds the midpoint. The animated cartoon serves as a reward. Average articulation scores in this phase turn out to be higher than those in any of the other phases. Table B–2 and Figure B–2 illustrate the data.

The study indicates that a novel, visually entertaining reward system positively affects the patient's performance when contrasted with a standard feedback signal, and points to a motivational element in the patient's performance. Go to Statistical Analysis for Example 2.

Table B–2. Patient's scores on Sentence Articulation in Baseline, First Intervention, Withdrawal, and Second Intervention Phases

Sentence Articulation Score	2 2 3 2 3 3 4 3 3 2	3 2 3 3 4 3 4 3 3 3	2 3 3 3 2 4 4 3 2 3	4 5 5 4 4 3 5 4 4 5
Trials	1 2 3 4 5 6 7 8 9 10	11 12 13 14 15 16 17 18 19 20	21 22 23 24 25 26 27 28 29 30	31 32 33 34 35 36 37 38 39 40
	Baseline (A_1)	Intervention (B_1)	Withdrawal (A_2)	Intervention (B_2)

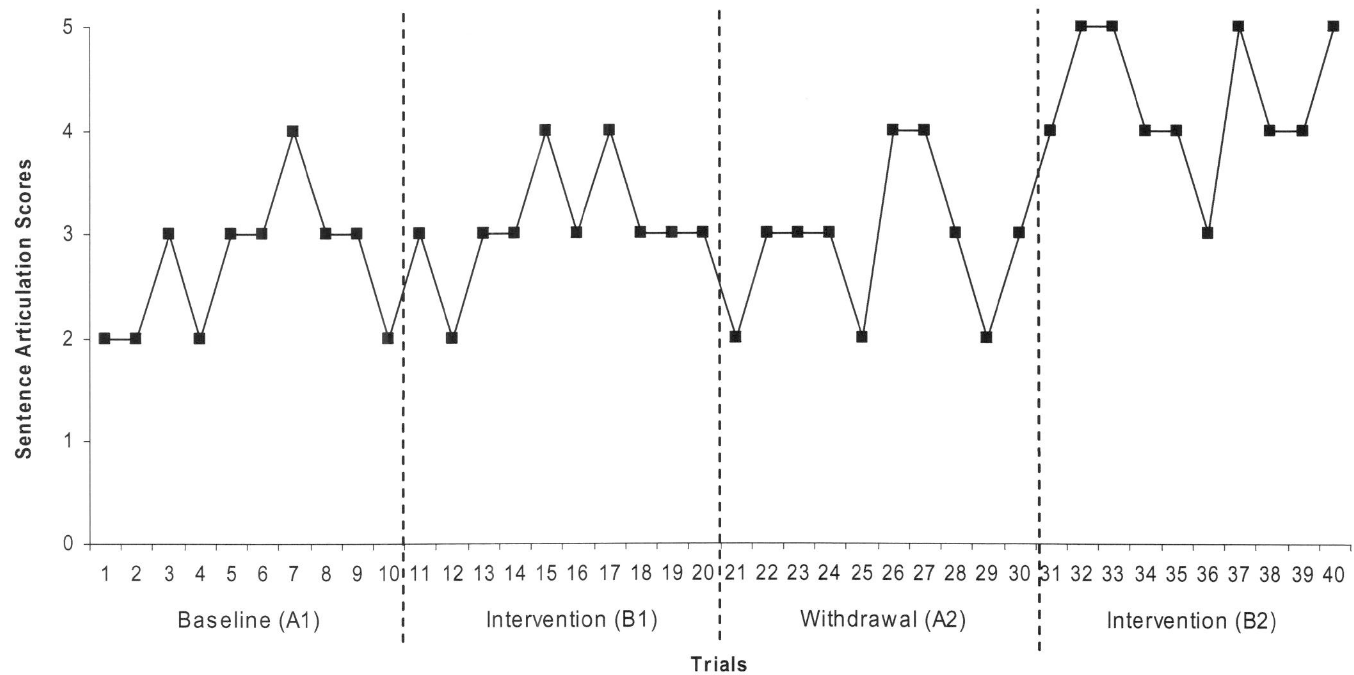

Figure B–2. Graphical illustration of patient's Sentence Articulation across each phase of the A-B–A-B study.

61

STATISTICAL ANALYSIS FOR EXAMPLE 1

Data from Table B–1: Patient's scores on sentence production—A-B-A-B Design.

A_1 = Baseline 1, B_1 = Intervention 1, A_2 = Withdrawal, B_2 = Intervention 2

Using the statistical software packages, like SPSS, SAS, MINITAB 14, and so forth, we can perform several analyses as follows.

1. Descriptive Statistics

A_1: MEAN = 5.10, MEDIAN = 5, SD = 1.20, $n = 10$
B_1: MEAN = 5.70, MEDIAN = 6, SD = 0.95, $n = 10$
A_2: MEAN = 5.40, MEDIAN = 5.50, SD = 1.17, $n = 10$
B_2: MEAN = 7.50, MEDIAN = 7.50, SD = 0.85, $n = 10$

Correlation Coefficients: r (A_1 and B_1) = −0.166, r (B_1 and A_2) = 0.219, r(A_2 and B_2) = −0.111

μ (A_1 and B_1) = 5.40, μ(B_1 and A_2) = 5.55, μ(A_2 and B_2) = 6.45

2. Analysis of Variance

(a) For the first three phases (A_1 and B_1 and A_2)

Sources	SS	df	MS = SS/df	F	p	Significance
Between	1.8	2	0.9	0.73	0.4923	Not significant
Within	33.4	27	1.237			

(b) For the second three phases (B_1 and A_2 and B_2)

Sources	SS	df	MS = SS/df	F	p	Significance
Between	25.8	2	12.9	12.9	<0.01	Highly significant
Within	27	27	1			

3. Autocorrelation Coefficients-Product-Moment lag-1

A_1: $r = 0.12, p = 0.75728$
B_1: $r = −0.375, p = 0.32$
A_2: $r = −0.110, p = 0.77797$
B_2: $r = −0.357, p = 0.3454$

4. Mann-Whitney U Test

(c) For the first two phases (A_1 and B_1)

   $U = 35.5$, $Z = 1.09$, $p > 0.05$ (Not significant)

(d) For the next two phases (B_1 and A_2)

   $U = 42.5$, $Z = 0.56$, $p > 0.05$ (Not significant)

(e) For the second three phases (A_2 and B_2)

   $U = 7.5$, $Z = 3.21$, $p < 0.01$ (Highly significant)

5. *t*-test

(f) For the first two phases (A_1 and B_1)

   $t(18) = 1.242$, $p = 0.230$ (Not significant)

(g) For the next two phases (B_1 and A_2)

   $t(18) = 0.628$, $p = 0.537$ (Not significant)

(h) For the second three phases (A_2 and B_2)

   $t(18) = 4.582$, $p = 0.000$ (Highly significant)

6. Time-Series Analysis

Phases	C	$Z = C/SE$	p-value	Significance
A_1	0.263	0.927	0.177	Not significant
B_1	0.382	1.346	0.089	Not significant
A_1 and B_1	0.342	1.610	0.053	Not significant
A_2	−0.088	−0.312	0.622	Not significant
B_1 and A_2	0.093	0.438	0.330	Not significant
B_2	−0.307	−1.082	0.860	Not significant
A_2 and B_2	0.413	1.948	0.025	Significant

Where $SE = SQR\,[(n-2)/(n+1)(n-1)]$, $C = 1-[\Sigma(X_i\text{-}X_{i+1})^2/2\Sigma(X\text{-}\mu)^2]$, and $Z = C/SE$

7. Bayesian Analysis

Hypothesis: H_o: No Effect, H_a: An Effect Exists

(i) For the first two phases (A_1 and B_1)

Data	$(X_i - X_{i+1})$	$(X_i - X_{i+1})^2$	$(X - \mu)$	$(X - \mu)^2$	Phases
4	−1	1	−1.4	1.96	A_1
5	0	0	−0.4	0.16	
5	−1	1	−0.4	0.16	
6	1	1	0.6	0.36	
5	−1	1	−0.4	0.16	
6	3	9	0.6	0.36	
3	−1	1	−2.4	5.76	
4	−2	4	−1.4	1.96	
6	−1	1	0.6	0.36	
7	1	1	1.6	2.56	
6	−1	1	0.6	0.36	B_1
7	0	0	1.6	2.56	
7	1	1	1.6	2.56	
6	1	1	0.6	0.36	
5	1	1	−0.4	0.16	
4	−2	4	−1.4	1.96	
6	1	1	0.6	0.36	
5	0	0	−0.4	0.16	
5	−1	1	−0.4	0.16	
6	—	—	0.6	0.36	
SUM (Σ)		30		22.8	

Therefore, we can obtain the values of C, SE, and Z (by the formulas shown under Time-Series Analysis) as follows.

$n = 20$, SE $= 0.212$, C $= 0.3421$, and Z $= 1.61$ ($p = 0.0537$ is also called "Likelihood").

Keep repeating this process, we eventually are able to calculate Likelihood, Bayes Factor (the ratio of likelihoods), and posterior probability of each consecutive phases (See Questions 34 and 36 in Part I for further details.)

The following table shows a summary of the results of each phase.

Phases	Hypothesis	Prior Probability	Likelihood	Bayes Factor (λ)	Prior × Likelihood	Posterior Probability	
A_1B_1	H_o	0.5	0.0537	0.05675	0.02685	0.0537	Moderate Treatment Effect*
	H_a	0.5	0.9463		0.47315	0.9463	
B_1A_2	H_o	0.0537	0.33	0.4925	0.017721	0.0272	Weak Withdrawal Effect**
	H_a	0.9463	0.67		0.634021	0.9728	
A_2B_2	H_o	0.0272	0.023	0.02354	0.0006256	0.000658	Moderate to Strong Treatment Effect***
	H_a	0.9728	0.977		0.9504256	0.999342	

*The strength of evidence during the first two phases showed that the first treatment is Moderate.

**The strength of evidence during the second two phases showed that the withdrawal effect is Weak, that is, the treatment is still effective during the period of withdrawal.

***The strength of evidence during the last two phases showed that the treatment is Very Effective after withdrawal phase.

8. Celeration Line

The following figures show the celeration line of this A-B-A-B Design. For further details, readers should review Question 12 in Part I.)

(Figure B–3, first two phases A_1B_1; Figure B–4, middle two phases B_1A_2; and Figure B–5, last two phases A_2B_2.)

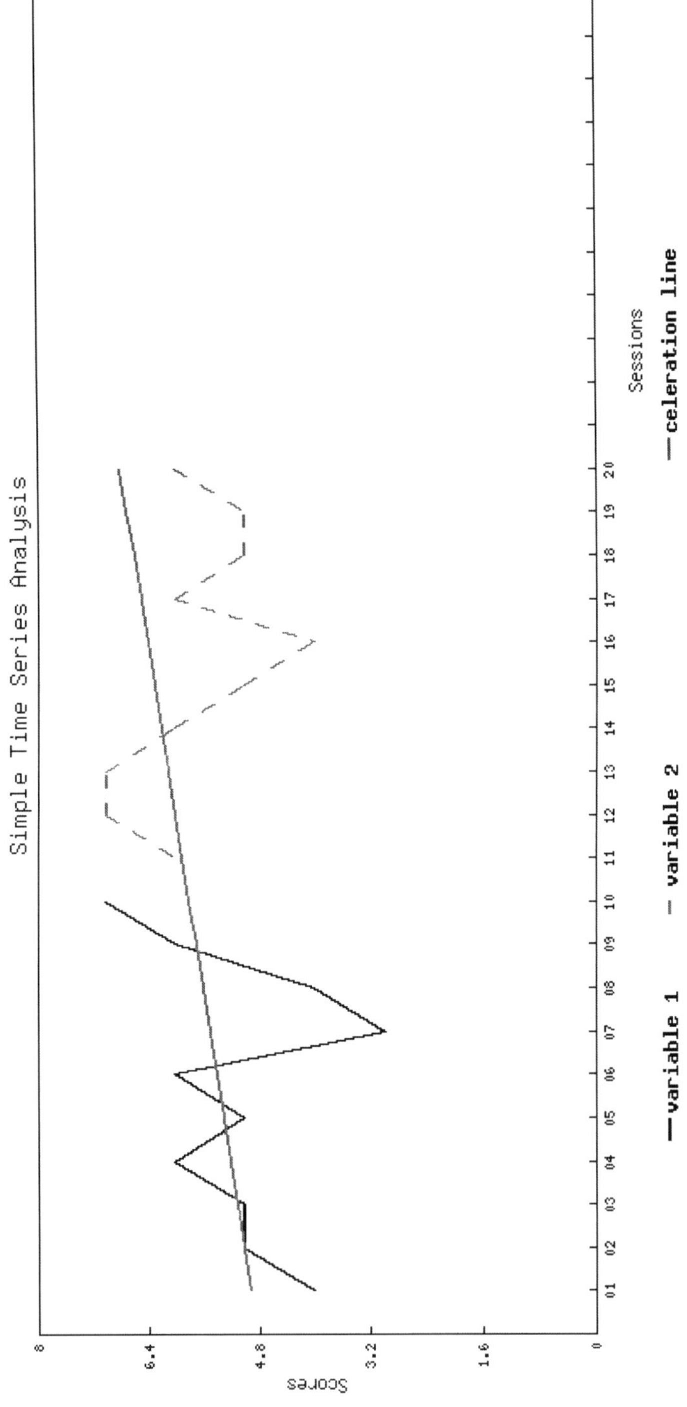

Figure B–3. First two phases A_1B_1 (A_1 = Variable 1, B_1 = Variable 2).

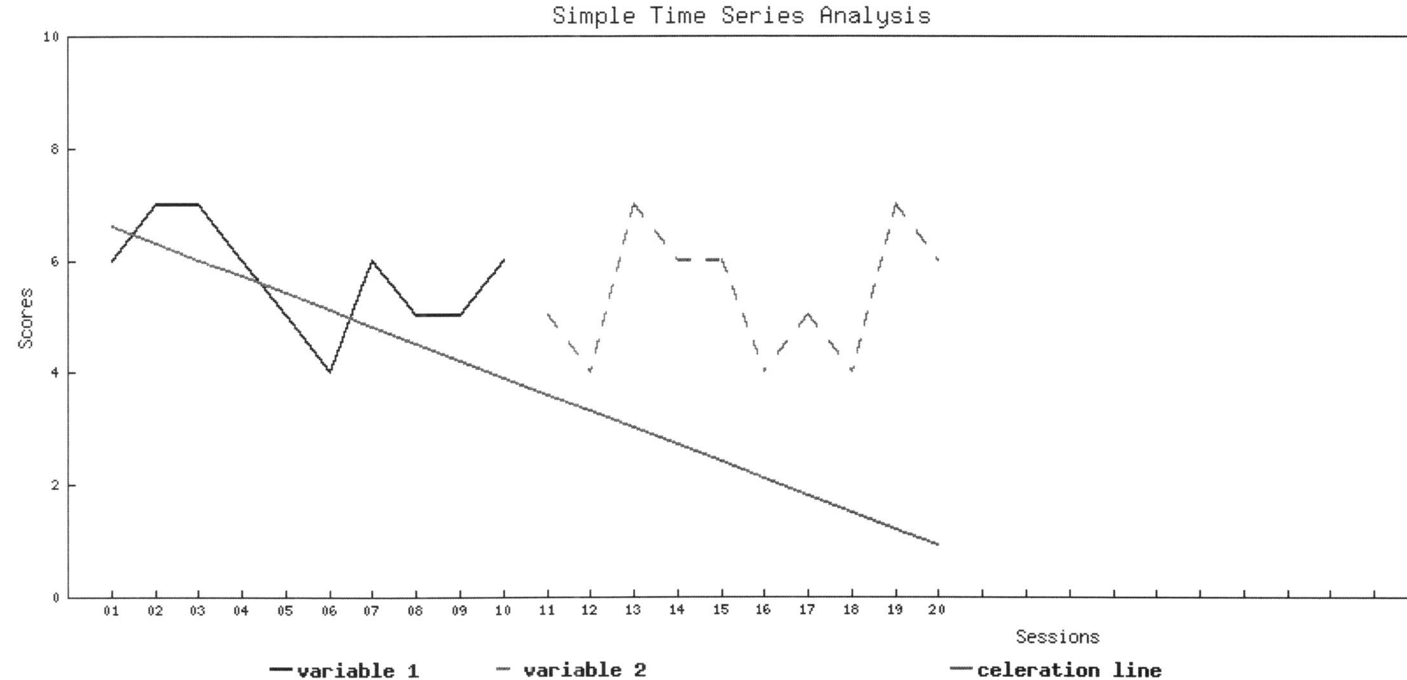

Figure B–4. Middle two phases B_1A_2 (B_1 = Variable 1, A_2 = Variable 2).

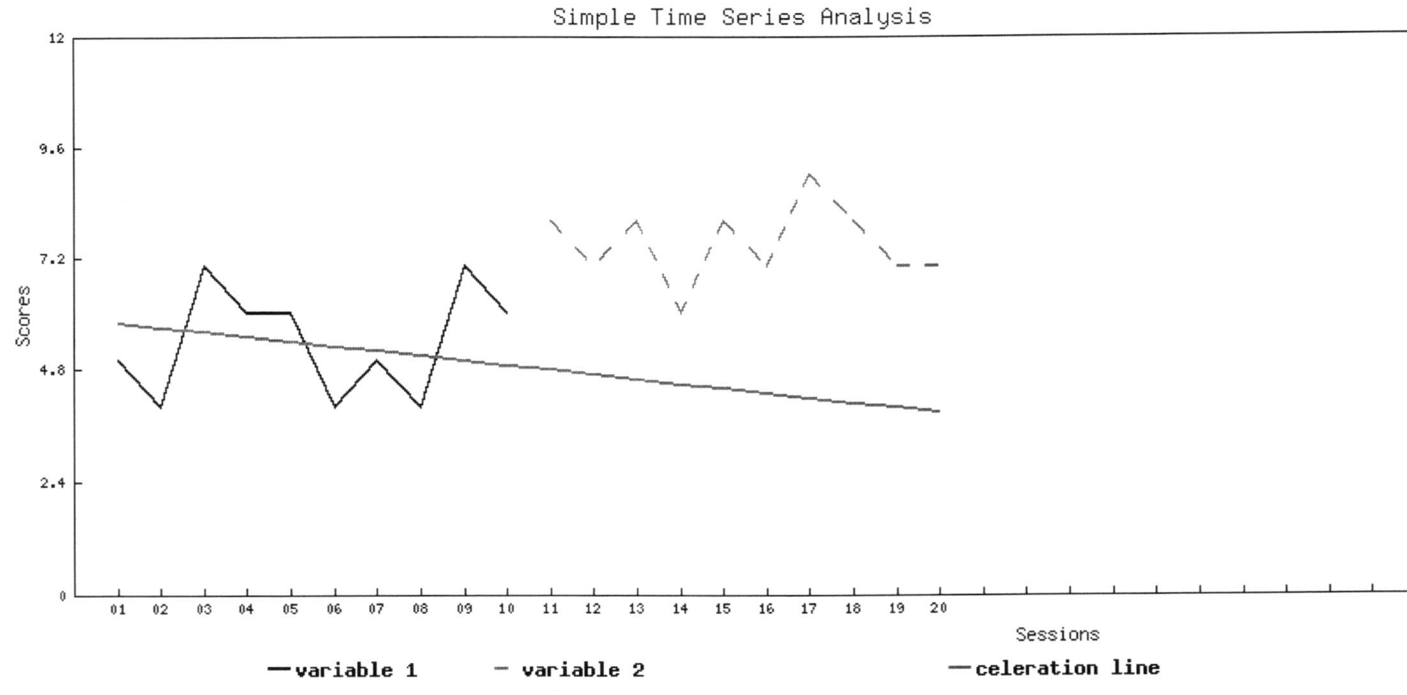

Figure B–5. Last two phases A_2B_2 (A_2 = Variable 1, B_2 = Variable 2).

9. χ^2 Analysis

Phases	Below (Undesired)*	Above (Desired)**
A_1	5	5
B_1	1	9

* and **: Below or Above the Celeration Line. See Part I for further details.

χ^2 ($n = 20$) = 3.809, p >0.05 (Not significant)

Phases	Below (Undesired)*	Above (Desired)**
B_1	3	7
A_2	2	8

* and **: Below or Above the Celeration Line. See Part I for further details.

χ^2 ($n = 20$) = 0.266, p >0.05 (Not significant).

Phases	Below (Undesired)*	Above (Desired)**
A_2	5	5
B_2	6	4

* and **: Below or Above the Celeration Line. See Part I for further details.

χ^2 ($n = 20$) = 0.202, p >0.05 (Not significant)

STATISTICAL ANALYSIS FOR EXAMPLE 2

Data from Table B–2: Patient's scores on sentence articulation—A-B-A-B Design.

A_1 = Baseline 1, B_1 = Intervention 1, A_2 = Withdrawal, B_2 = Intervention 2

Using the statistical software packages, like SPSS, SAS, MINITAB 14, and so forth, we can perform several analyses as follows.

1. Descriptive Statistics

A_1: MEAN = 2.70, MEDIAN = 3, SD = 0.674, n = 10
B_1: MEAN = 3.10, MEDIAN = 3, SD = 0.567, n = 10
A_2: MEAN = 2.90, MEDIAN = 3, SD = 0.737, n = 10
B_2: MEAN = 4.30, MEDIAN = 4, SD = 0.674, n = 10

Correlation Coefficients: r (A_1 and B_1) = 0.667, r (B_1 and A_2) = 0.026, r (A_2 and B_2) = 0.066

μ (A_1 and B_1) = 2.90, μ(B_1 and A_2) = 3, μ(A_2 and B_2) = 3.65

2. Analysis of Variance

(a) For the first three phases (A_1 and B_1 and A_2)

Sources	SS	df	MS = SS/df	F	p	Significance
Between	0.8	2	0.4	0.908	0.4155	Not significant
Within	11.9	27	0.441			

(b) For the second three phases (B_1 and A_2 and B_2)

Sources	SS	df	MS = SS/df	F	p	Significance
Between	11.467	2	5.733	13.008	<0.01	Highly significant
Within	11.9	27	0.441			

3. Autocorrelation Coefficients-Product-Moment lag-1

A_1: r = 0.156, p = 0.68809
B_1: r = −0.038, p = 0.92174
A_2: r = 0.00, p = 1.00
B_2: r = −0.176, p = 0.64912

4. Mann-Whitney U Test

    (c) For the first two phases (A_1 and B_1)

        $U = 51.0$, $Z = 0.07$, $p > 0.05$ (Not significant)

    (d) For the next two phases (B_1 and A_2)

        $U = 59.5$, $Z = 0.71$, $p > 0.05$ (Not significant)

    (e) For the second three phases (A_2 and B_2)

        $U = 9.5$, $Z = 3.06$, $p < 0.01$ (Highly significant)

5. *t*-test

    (f) For the first two phases (A_1 and B_1)

        $t(18) = 1.434$, $p = 0.168$ (Not significant)

    (g) For the next two phases (B_1 and A_2)

        $t(18) = 0.679$, $p = 0.505$ (Not significant)

    (h) For the second three phases (A_2 and B_2)

        $t(18) = 4.427$, $p = 0.000$ (Highly significant)

6. Time-Series Analysis

Phases	C	$Z = C/SE$	p-value	Significance
A_1	0.268	0.943	0.172	Not significant
B_1	−0.034	−0.121	0.548	Not significant
A_1 and B_1	0.166	0.784	0.216	Not significant
A_2	0.081	0.287	0.387	Not significant
B_1 and A_2	0.000	0.000	0.500	Not significant
B_2	−0.097	−0.343	0.634	Not significant
A_2 and B_2	0.494	2.329	0.009	Highly Significant

Where $SE = SQR\ [(n-2)/(n+1)(n-1)]$, $C = 1 - [\Sigma(X_i - X_{i+1})^2 / 2\Sigma(X - \mu)^2]$, and $Z = C/SE$

7. Bayesian Analysis

Hypothesis: H_o: No Effect, H_a: An Effect Exists

(i) For the first two phases (A_1 and B_1)

Data	(X_i-X_{i+1})	$(X_i-X_{i+1})^2$	$(X-\mu)$	$(X-\mu)^2$	Phases
2	0	0	−0.9	0.81	A_1
2	−1	1	−0.9	0.81	
3	1	1	0.1	0.01	
2	−1	1	−0.9	0.81	
3	0	0	0.1	0.01	
3	−1	1	0.1	0.01	
4	1	1	1.1	1.21	
3	0	0	0.1	0.01	
3	1	1	0.1	0.01	
2	−1	1	−0.9	0.81	
3	1	1	0.1	0.01	B_1
2	−1	1	−0.9	0.81	
3	0	0	0.1	0.01	
3	−1	1	0.1	0.01	
4	1	1	1.1	1.21	
3	−1	1	0.1	0.01	
4	1	1	1.1	1.21	
3	0	0	0.1	0.01	
3	0	0	0.1	0.01	
3	—	—	0.1	0.01	
SUM (Σ)		13		7.8	

Therefore, we can obtain the values of C, SE, and Z (by the formulas shown under Time-Series Analysis) as follows.

$n = 20$, SE = 0.212, C = 0.166, and Z = 0.80 ($p = 0.2119$ is also called "Likelihood").

Keep repeating this process, we eventually are able to calculate Likelihood, Bayes Factor (the ratio of likelihoods), and posterior probability of each consecutive phases (See Questions 34 and 36 in Part I for further details.)

The following table shows a summary of the results of each phase.

Phases	Hypothesis	Prior Probability	Likelihood	Bayes Factor (λ)	Prior × Likelihood	Posterior Probability	
A_1B_1	H_o	0.5	0.2119	0.2689	0.10595	0.2119	Weak Treatment Effect*
	H_a	0.5	0.7881		0.39405	0.7881	
B_1A_2	H_o	0.2119	0.5	1.00	0.10595	0.2119	Weak Withdrawal Effect**
	H_a	0.7881	0.5		0.39405	0.7881	
A_2B_2	H_o	0.2119	0.01	0.0101	0.002119	0.0027	Moderate to Strong Treatment Effect***
	H_a	0.7881	0.99		0.780219	0.9973	

*The strength of evidence during the first two phases showed that the first treatment is Weak.

**The strength of evidence during the second two phases showed that the withdrawal effect is Weak, that is, the treatment is still somewhat effective during the period of withdrawal.

***The strength of evidence during the last two phases showed that the treatment is Very Effective after withdrawal phase.

8. Celeration Line

The following figures show the celeration line of this A-B-A-B Design. (For further details, readers should review Question 12 in Part I.)

(Figure B-6, first two phases A_1B_1; Figure B-7, middle two phases B_1A_2; Figure B-8, last two phases A_2B_2.)

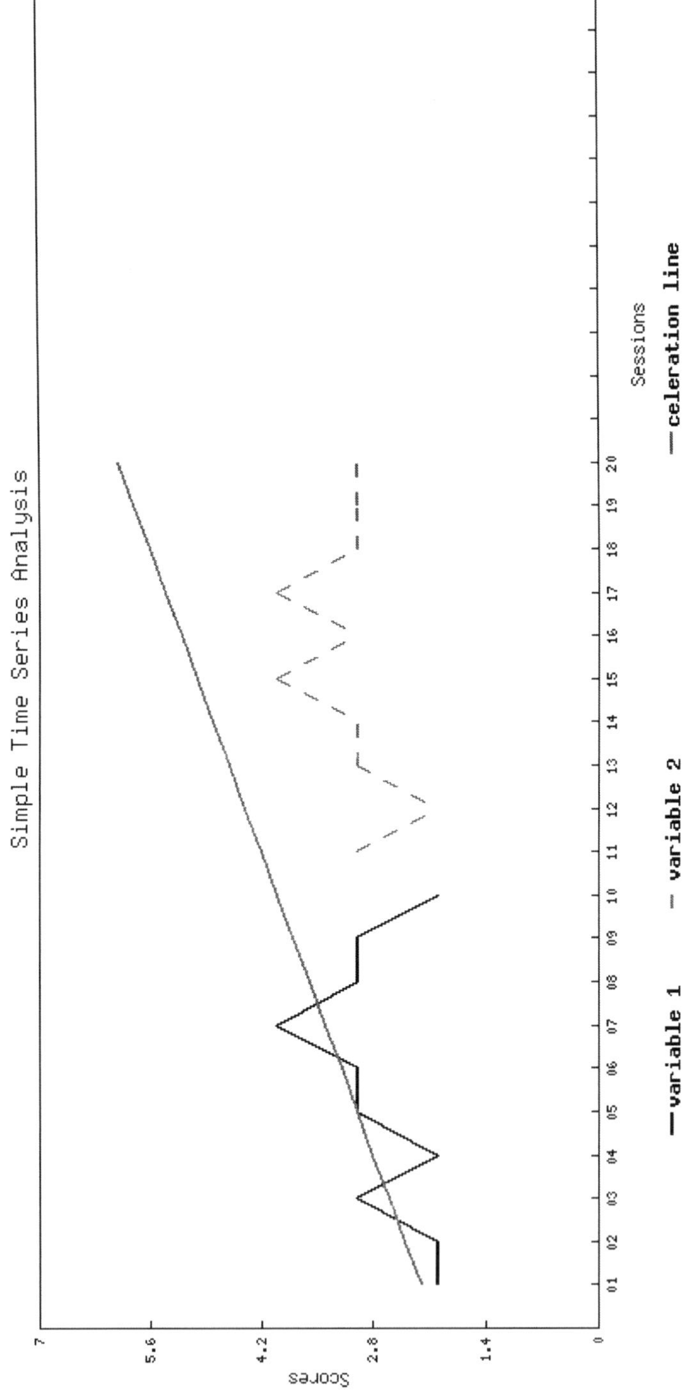

Figure B–6. First two phases A_1B_1 (A_1 = Variable 1, B_1 = Variable 2).

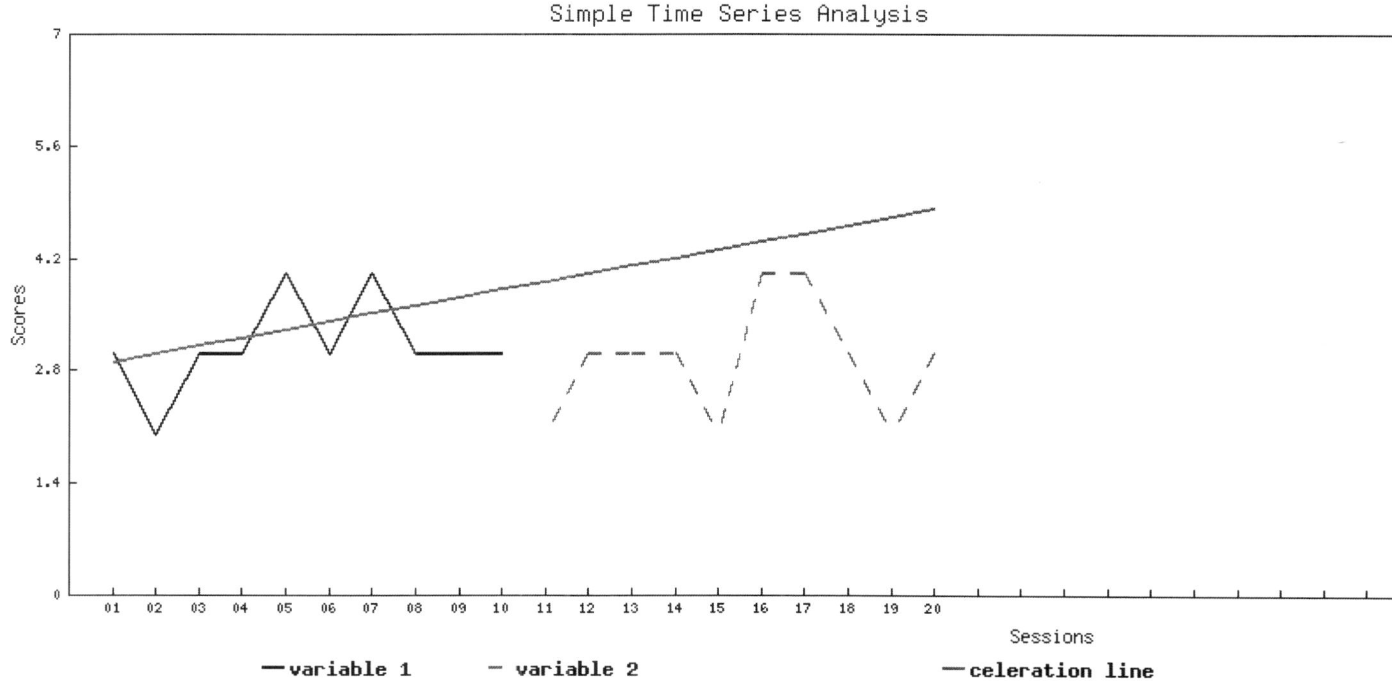

Figure B–7. Middle two phases B_1A_2 (B_1 = Variable 1, A_2 = Variable 2).

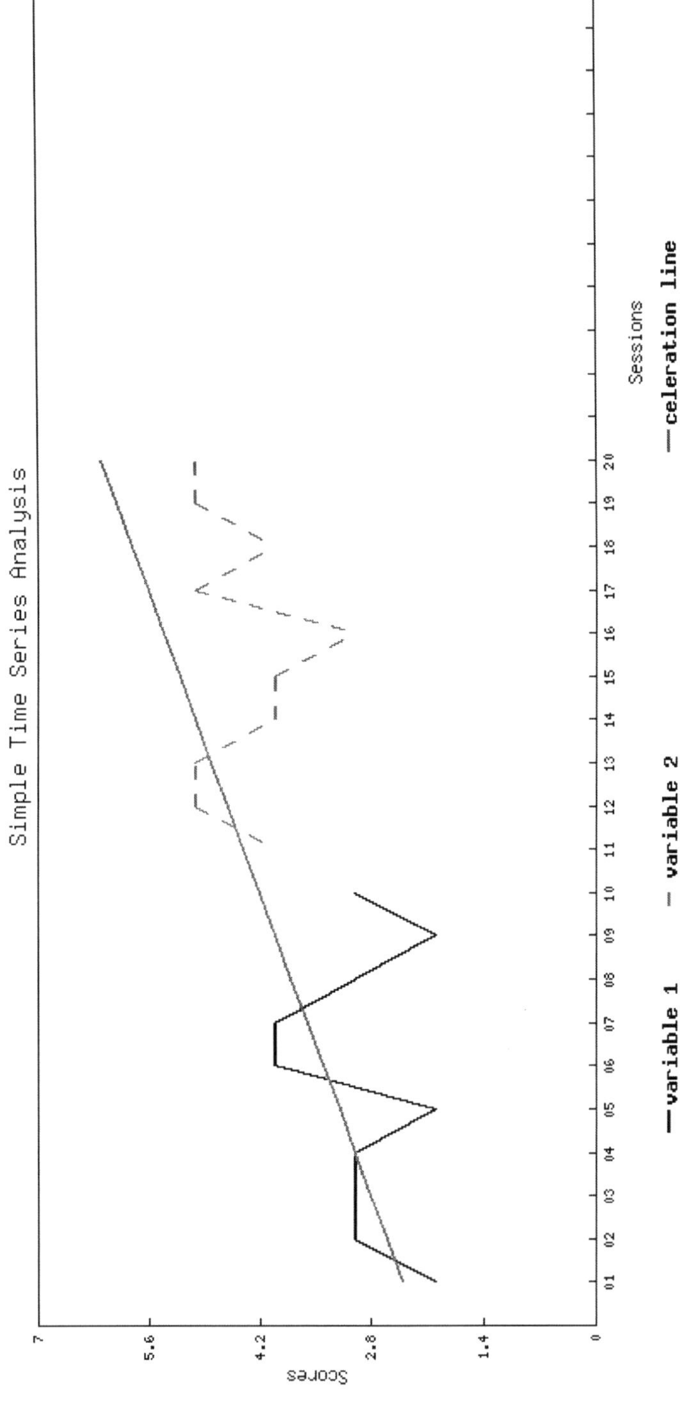

Figure B–8. Last two phases A_2B_2 (A_2 = Variable 1, B_2 = Variable 2).

9. χ^2 Analysis

Phases	Below (Undesired)*	Above (Desired)**
A_1	5	5
B_1	6	4

* and **: Below or Above the Celeration Line. See Part I for further details.

χ^2 ($n = 20$) = 0.202, p >0.05 (Not significant)

Phases	Below (Undesired)*	Above (Desired)**
B_1	4	6
A_2	9	1

* and **: Below or Above the Celeration Line. See Part I for further details.

χ^2 ($n = 20$) = 5.494, p <0.05 (Significant)

Phases	Below (Undesired)*	Above (Desired)**
A_2	5	5
B_2	10	0

* and **: Below or Above the Celeration Line. See Part I for further details.

χ^2 ($n = 20$) = 6.666, p <0.01 (Highly significant)

SECTION C

Single Subject Designs in Clinical and Rehabilitation Psychology

Overview

Over the past 25 years, a clear case has been made for the utility of single subjects designs in clinical, counseling, and rehabilitation psychology. The use of single subject designs as a convenient statistical tool and as a way of embracing the scientist-practitioner model has found its way in to many areas of clinical psychology, cognitive and psychodynamic interventions, and psychiatric and substance abuse treatment. The uniqueness of these clinical contexts and the particular constraints found within them provide great opportunity for single subject design applications. Various supporting arguments have been put forth in making the case for single subject design application in these clinical realms (Barlow, Hayes, & Nelson, 1984; Galassi & Gersh, 1993; McReynolds & Thompson, 1986): The daily reality of the clinical environment and its time constraints are not necessarily conducive to large-scale controlled experi-ments; clinicians are not full-time scientists and often cannot afford the time for conventional controlled studies. The individual client focus of the typical clinician gives many causes for single subject designs; for example, it allows for a patient's change or progress to be analyzed over a course of treatment. Within a group of patients sharing the same diagnosis, there is often wide variation of the clinical profile. Here, the single subject design is ideally suited to profiling these individual cases. In the context of clinical practice, a single subject design can be an effective support tool in generating hypotheses, and a clinician can apply these designs without having to labor over a great deal of statistical theory. A clinician can use the design to carry out a quick test of a new remedial measure. Altogether, single subject designs used in the context of clinical and counseling psychology promote data collection, better selection and guidance of counseling interventions, and foster stronger relationships between clinical methods and outcomes.

Examples of Research Studies in Clinical and Rehabilitation Psychology Where Single Subject Designs Have Been Employed

The very wide variety of applications for single subject designs in clinical and rehabilitation psychology is clearly tied to the breadth of these clinical fields. For a survey of the many research questions in these fields that can be addressed with single subject designs, see Galassi and Gersh (1993) and Callahan and Barisa (2005). Research questions can range, for example, from assessing the efficacy of a training program for school psychologists (Maher, 1985) or the efficacy of psychoanalytic interventions (Fonagy & Moran, 1990) to measurement of the success in treatment outcomes in patients with schizophrenia (Iyer, Rothman, Vogler, & Spaulding, 2005). We consider three examples.

A powerful illustration of the utility of single subject designs in the study of severe psychiatric illness was made by Kupper and Tschacher (2002). The researchers were interested in profiling symptom development during acute episodes of schizophrenia, an area that was reported to be poorly understood. They used a time series to examine symptom trajectories in 46 patients that ranged in terms of schizophrenia subtypes and symptoms. The time series was based on daily observations of the "psychoticity," "excitement," and "withdrawal" symptoms in each of the patients during the course of treatment. This would provide a view to the symptom trajectories, which symptoms may be interdependent and during which phase, and so forth. Many patterns emerged from the results. For example, the symptoms of psychosis showed relative independence from the other symptoms in terms of their change over time, but they also showed a relationship to the level of initial withdrawal symptoms.

Clare, Wilson, Carter, and Hodges (2003) described a single case study that looked at the role of particular cognitive interventions in improving the memory capacity of a patient with early-stage Alzheimer's disease. Among the patient's cognitive difficulties was a difficulty in remembering the names of people familiar to him. The study involved baseline, intervention, postintervention, and follow-up phases. The researchers' training methods (intervention) involved specific memory strategies such as mnemonics and repeated stimulus presentation. The patient was trained on a task involving pictures of familiar people and their names. The patient's baseline naming score was close to zero. Postintervention scores and scores at 1- and 3-month follow-up periods (when the patient was practicing the naming strategies at home) were above 80%. Follow-up at 6 months, after the patient stopped the naming practice, showed a drop in his score but the score was still above the baseline score. Through a single case illustration, the study pointed to the potential specific memory exercises in aiding patients with early-stage Alzheimer's disease.

Patients with memory deficits secondary to brain insults often lack an awareness of the deficits, and such was the subject of a study by Rebmann and Hannon (1995). The authors carried out single subject studies on three patients who showed a lack of awareness of their memory deficits while recovering from brain injury. An A-B design was used. The researchers first measured the patients' unawareness of memory deficits (baseline) by using a memory test and then asking the patients to describe their scores, over 4 to 5 baseline sessions. This was followed by similar testing but accompanied with behavioral modification measures that involved visual and verbal feedback and positive reinforcement. Six to eight of these treatment sessions were applied. Reinforcers in the form of verbal praise and lottery tickets were given at the end of each treatment session if the patient showed a decrease in memory unawareness. The treatment and the assessment of the treatment therefore occurred in the same phase (B) of the study. All subjects showed improvement during the treatment sessions but rate of improvement followed a different path for each subject, and one patient's improvement was far less than that of the other two. One patient, for example, showed step improvement in the second treatment session whereas another showed improvement only in the fifth session. At the very least, the results reasserted the possibility of using behavioral modification to counter patients' lack of memory deficits.

In the three examples described above, the single subject methodology was optimally suited to the research question or context. In the study by Kupper and Tschacher, multiple sets of data gathered through a time series approach yielded dynamic patterns in symptom profiles, patterns that would have been very difficult to infer without the time series structure. The study by Clare, et al (2003) involved customized training methods, the patient's practice at home, and three follow-up sessions. This level of attention would not be feasible with a large sample set, especially in the short term. This study simply sought to evaluate the effectiveness of certain cognitive strategies that patients with Alzheimer's disease and their family members could implement to improve patients memory in certain domains. The affirmative results offered some validation for the rehabilitative strategy employed. That effectiveness of the strategy was all the study sought to investigate and the single subject design was an expedient way to carry out the investigation. The feedback and reinforcement in the behavioral modification study by Rebmann and Hannon (1995), required a complex engagement of steps and contingent measures by the clinicians in the course of behavioral modification. Again, a single subject design enabled the researchers to gauge the promise of the technique, and the results supported further investigation.

Examples of Data Sets (two hypothetical cases)

We consider two cases, first, A-B-C design[1] (A followed by two successive treatments B and C) and second, A-B design with two dependent measures.

Example 1

A patient with a memory disorder undergoes clinical assessment. The patient's memory deficits are found to be primarily with common objects. The examiner then wishes to make a quick assessment as to whether the patient's difficulties with naming common objects can be improved with phonemic or semantic cues about the objects. Memory for common objects is then tested (baseline) with a special pictorial test that involves 15 trials. Each trial is scored on 3 points—dependent on speed, accuracy, and completeness of the response. Following this baseline phase, the clinician adds 5 more trials to the test, randomizes the entire set of trials, and divides them into two sets of 10 trials. The treatment session follows. One set of 10 trials are presented and after each prompt for a name, the pa-

---

[1]A potential limitation of this design is confounding influence of the first treatment (B) on the second treatment (C) due to a carryover effect.

tient is given phonemic cue for the name. In the second set of 10 trials, the patient is given a semantic cue for the name. Results indicate that both kinds of cues improve the patient's naming compared to baseline levels. It also shows that semantic cues improve the patient's naming more than phonemic cues. Table C-1 and Figure C-1 illustrate the data.

The clinician applied a single subject design to get a quick gauge of the kinds of naming cues that best aid the subject's word finding difficulties. Naming of common objects was best aided with semantic cues. With such data in hand, the clinician can look for further relationships between cue types and types of anomia in individual patients. Go to Statistical Analysis for Example 1.

Example 2

A patient is diagnosed with social phobia (an anxiety disorder). The patient is referred to a clinician who specializes in treating social phobia with a combination of cognitive therapy and biofeedback. The patient and the clinician opt for a program with a fixed number of sessions over a 4-week period due to insurance limitations. In the first 10 sessions, baseline measures of anxiety are obtained using a rating scale of the patient's responses to a test that involves viewing scenes of various social settings. The scale ranges from 1 to 20, 1 indicating very low anxiety level. Baseline anxiety is also measured with biofeedback data on the patient's muscle tension, skin response, and heart rate. The three biofeedback scores are averaged and are also expressed on a 1 to 20-point scale. Anxiety baseline scores on both measures are found to be high. Nine sessions of treatment then follow. Treatment sessions involve the same setup as the baseline assessment phase (tests of social phobia and biofeedback indicators) but also include teaching the patient's cognitive awareness and cognitive techniques, following the patient's responses to the test stimuli. Over the course of the nine treatment sessions, the patient's scores on the tests of social phobia gradually drops to lower levels. The biofeedback scores also drop gradually. Table C-2 and Figure C-2 illustrate the data.

The single subject design enabled the clinician to (1) confirm very soon after baseline assessment that the interventions were associating with in a decrease of the subject's anxiety levels, and (2) test the efficacy of two treatment modalities. The clinician has established a model for applying the treatment types over a short period to achieve remedial effects in a patient. Go to Statistical Analysis for Example 2.

(In the analysis that follows, the raw scores from Tables C-1 and C-2 are converted into decimal form. In order to perform the Bayesian Approach with beta distribution for the analysis and interpretation of single subject data, all raw scores must be converted into their decimal equivalent.

Table C–1. Patient's scores in naming common objects, over 15 baseline trials, 10 trials with phonemic cues, and 10 trials with semantic cues

Score	1	0	0	1	2	1	0	0	0	3	1	0	0	1	2	2	1	2	0	3	2	2	3	0	1	3	3	2	3	1	2	3	2	3	3
Trials	1	2	3	4	5	6	7	8	9	10	11	12	13	14	15	16	17	18	19	20	21	22	23	24	25	26	27	28	29	30	31	32	33	34	35
	No Cues															Phonemic Cues										Semantic Cues									
	(Baseline)															(Treatment)																			

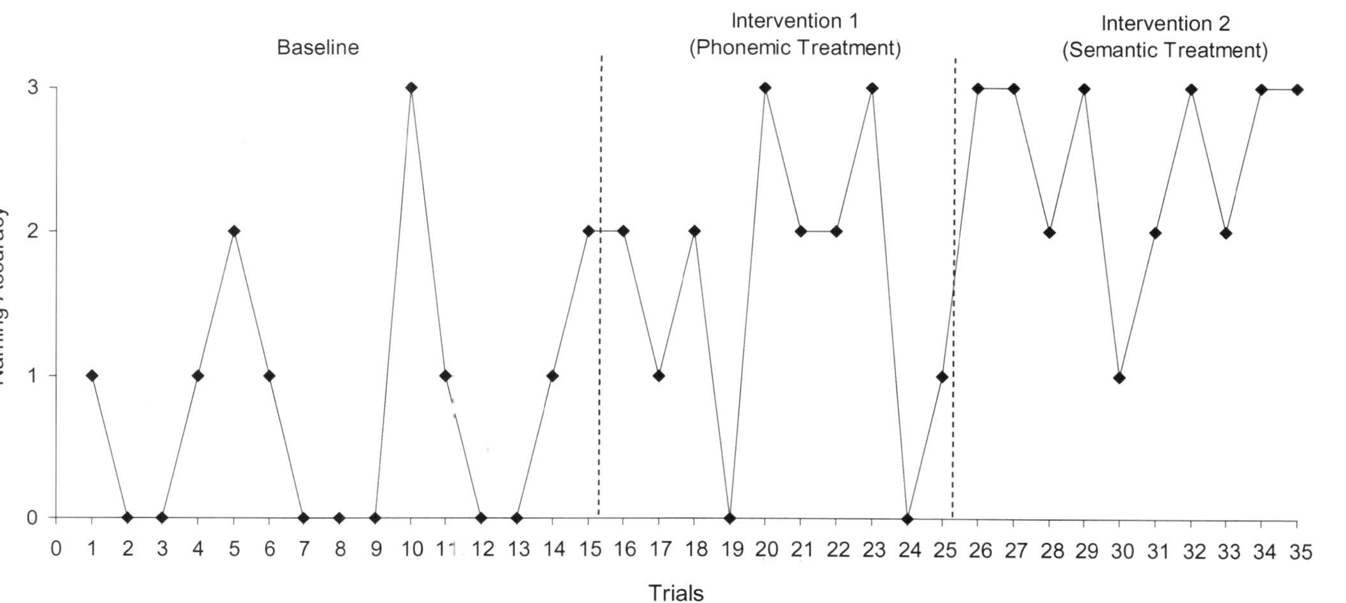

Figure C–1. Graphical illustration of patient's naming accuracy over 15 baseline trials, 10 trials with phonemic cues, and 10 trials with semantic cues.

Table C–2. Patient's anxiety levels (social phobia and biofeedback scores) at 10 baseline sessions and 9 treatment sessions

Biofeedback Average	10	10	11	12	13	12	10	9	13	11	8	7	7	7	6	7	5	4	4
Social Phobia Level	16	15	17	17	16	15	16	15	16	15	14	12	10	8	8	8	7	8	7
Sessions	1	2	3	4	5	6	7	8	9	10	11	12	13	14	15	16	17	18	19
	Baseline										Treatment								

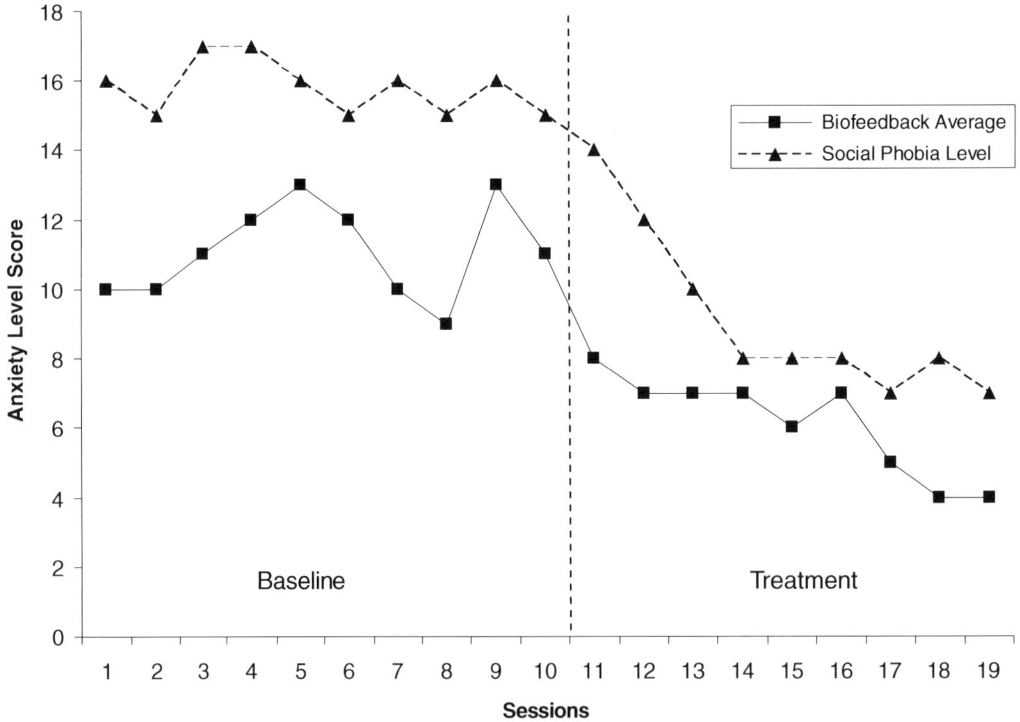

Figure C–2. Graphical illustration of patient's anxiety levels during baseline and treatment sessions.

STATISTICAL ANALYSIS FOR EXAMPLE 1
(Clinical and Rehabilitation Psychology)

Data from Table C–1: Patient's scores in naming common objects—a modified (a.k.a A-B-C design) A-B Design.

A_1 = Baseline 1, B_1 = Intervention 1

Using the statistical software packages, like SPSS, SAS, MINITAB 14, and so forth, we can perform several analyses as follows. For this particular design, we combine two successive treatments B and C together, therefore, let A_1 be a baseline and B_1 be a treatment.

1. Descriptive Statistics

A_1: MEAN = 0.80, MEDIAN = 1, SD = 0.941, n =15
B_1: MEAN = 2.05, MEDIAN = 2, SD = 0.998, n = 20

Correlation Coefficients: r (A_1 and B_1) = −0.214

μ (A_1 and B_1) = 1.5143

2. Analysis of Variance

(a) For the two phases (A_1 and B_1)

Sources	SS	df	MS = SS/df	*F*	*p*	Significance
Between	13.393	1	13.393	14.098	<0.01	Highly significant
Within	31.35	33	0.95			

3. Autocorrelation Coefficients-Product-Moment lag-1

A_1: r = 0.098, p = 0.73719
B_1: r = −0.108, p = 0.65899

4. Mann-Whitney U Test

(b) For the two phases (A_1 and B_1)
   U = 76.0, Z = 2.46, p <0.05 (Significant)

5. *t*-test

(c) For the two phases (A_1 and B_1)
   t(33) = 3.754, p = 0.000 (Highly significant)

6. Time-Series Analysis

Phases	C	$Z = C/SE$	p-value	Significance
A_1	0.153	0.636	0.262	Not significant
B_1	−0.081	−0.385	0.649	Not significant
A_1 and B_1	0.307	1.870	0.030	Significant

Where SE = SQR $[(n-2)/(n+1)(n-1)]$, C = $1-[\Sigma(X_i-X_{i+1})^2/2\Sigma(X-\mu)^2]$, and Z = C/SE

7. Bayesian Analysis

Hypothesis: H_o: No Effect, H_a: An Effect Exists

(d) For the first two phases (A_1 and B_1)

Data	(X_i-X_{i+1})	$(X_i-X_{i+1})^2$	$(X-\mu)$	$(X-\mu)^2$	Phases
1	1	1	−0.5143	0.2645	A_1
0	0	0	−1.5143	2.293	
0	−1	1	−1.5143	2.293	
1	−1	1	−0.5143	0.2645	
2	1	1	0.4857	0.236	
1	1	1	−0.5143	0.2645	
0	0	0	−1.5143	2.293	
0	0	0	−1.5143	2.293	
0	−3	9	−1.5143	2.293	
3	2	4	1.4857	2.207	
1	1	1	−0.5143	0.2645	
0	0	0	−1.5143	2.293	
0	−1	1	−1.5143	2.293	
1	−1	1	−0.5143	0.2645	
2	0	0	0.4857	0.236	
2	1	1	0.4857	0.236	B_1
1	−1	1	−0.5143	0.2645	
2	2	4	0.4857	0.236	
0	−3	9	−1.5143	2.293	
3	1	1	1.4857	2.207	

Data	(X_i-X_{i+1})	$(X_i-X_{i+1})^2$	$(X-\mu)$	$(X-\mu)^2$	Phases
2	0	0	0.4857	0.236	B_1
2	−1	1	0.4857	0.236	
3	3	9	1.4857	2.207	
0	−1	1	−1.5143	2.293	
1	−2	4	−0.5143	0.2645	
3	0	0	1.4857	2.207	
3	1	1	1.4857	2.207	
2	−1	1	0.4857	0.236	
3	2	4	1.4857	2.207	
1	−1	1	−0.5143	0.2645	
2	−1	1	0.4857	0.236	
3	1	1	1.4857	2.207	
2	−1	1	0.4857	0.236	
3	0	0	1.4857	2.207	
3	—	—	1.4857	2.207	
SUM (Σ)		62		44.74	

Therefore, we can obtain the values of C, SE, and Z (by the formulas shown under Time-Series Analysis) as follows.

$n = 35$, SE = 0.1642, C = 0.3071, and Z = 1.87 ($p = 0.030$ is also called "Likelihood").

Keep repeating this process, we eventually are able to calculate Likelihood, Bayes Factor (the ratio of likelihoods), and posterior probability of each consecutive phases (See Questions 34 and 36 in Part I for further details.)

The following table shows a summary of the results of each phase.

Phases	Hypothesis	Prior Probability	Likelihood	Bayes Factor (λ)	Prior × Likelihood	Posterior Probability	
A_1B_1	H_o	0.5	0.030	0.0309	0.015	0.030	Moderate to Strong Treatment Effect*
	H_a	0.5	0.970		0.485	0.970	

*The strength of evidence during the first two phases showed that the first treatment is Moderate to Strong.

8. Celeration Line

Figure C–3 (first two phases A_1B_1) is the celeration line of this A-B-A-B Design. (For further details, readers should review Question 12 in Part I.)

9. χ^{-2} Analysis

Phases	Below (Undesired)*	Above (Desired)**
A_1	7	8
B_1	15	5

* and **: Below or Above the Celeration Line. See Part I for further details.

χ^{-2} $(n = 35) = 2.947, p > 0.05$ (Not significant)

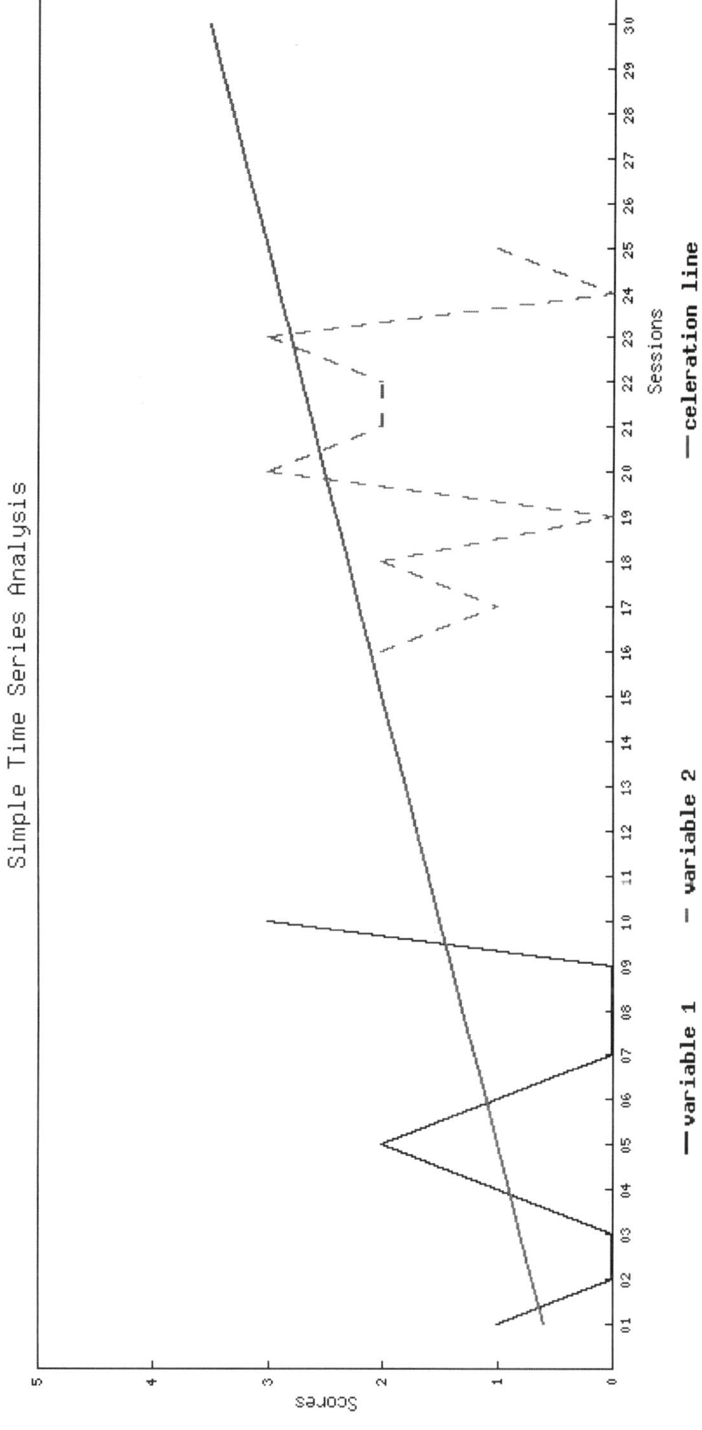

Figure C–3. First two phases A_1B_1 (A_1 = Variable 1, B_1 = Variable 2).

STATISTICAL ANALYSIS FOR EXAMPLE 2
(Clinical and Rehabilitation Psychology)

Data from Table C–2: Patient's anxiety levels (Biofeedback Scores)—A-B Design.

A_1 = Baseline 1, B_1 = Intervention 1

Using the statistical software packages, like SPSS, SAS, MINITAB 14, and so forth, we can perform several analyses as follows.

1. Descriptive Statistics

A_1: MEAN = 10.33, MEDIAN = 10, SD = 0.577, $n = 3$
B_1: MEAN = 6.11, MEDIAN = 7, SD = 1.452, $n = 9$

Correlation Coefficients: r (A_1 and B_1) = 0.624

μ (A_1 and B_1) = 7.17

2. Analysis of Variance

(e) For the two phases (A_1 and B_1)

Sources	SS	df	MS = SS/df	F	p	Significance
Between	40.111	1	40.111	22.848	<0.01	Highly significant
Within	17.556	10	1.756			

3. Mann-Whitney U Test

(f) For the first two phases (A_1 and B_1)

U = 0.00, Z = 2.49, p <0.05 (Significant)

4. t-test

(g) For the first two phases (A_1 and B_1)

$t(10)$ = 4.779, p = 0.000 (Highly significant)

5. Time-Series Analysis

Phases	C	$Z = C/SE$	p-value	Significance
A_1	0.249	0.707	0.239	Not significant
B_1	0.763	2.579	0.005	Highly significant
A_1 and B_1	0.843	3.191	0.001	Highly significant

Where SE = SQR $[(n-2)/(n+1)(n-1)]$, C = $1-[\Sigma(X_i-X_{i+1})^2/2\Sigma(X-\mu)^2]$, and Z = C/SE

6. Bayesian Analysis

Hypothesis: H_0: No Effect, H_a: An Effect Exists

(h) For the first two phases (A_1 and B_1)

Data	(X_i-X_{i+1})	$(X_i-X_{i+1})^2$	$(X-\mu)$	$(X-\mu)^2$	Phases
10	0	0	2.83	8	A_1
10	−1	1	2.83	8	
11	3	9	3.83	14.67	
8	1	1	0.83	0.69	B_1
7	0	0	−0.17	0.0289	
7	0	0	−0.17	0.0289	
7	1	1	−0.17	0.0289	
6	−1	1	−1.17	1.37	
7	2	4	−0.17	0.0289	
5	1	1	−2.17	4.71	
4	0	0	−3.17	10.05	
4	—	—	−3.17	10.05	
SUM (Σ)		18		57.6556	

Therefore, we can obtain the values of C, SE, and Z (by the formulas shown under Time-Series Analysis) as follows.

n =12, SE = 0.264, C = 0.8439, and Z = 3.191 (p = 0.001 is also called "Likelihood").

Keep repeating this process, we eventually are able to calculate Likelihood, Bayes Factor (the ratio of likelihoods), and posterior probability of each consecutive phases (See Questions 34 and 36 in Part I for further details.)

The following table shows a summary of the results of each phase.

Phases	Hypothesis	Prior Probability	Likelihood	Bayes Factor (λ)	Prior × Likelihood	Posterior Probability	
A_1B_1	H_o	0.5	0.001	0.001	0.0005	0.001	Strong to Very Strong Treatment Effect*
	H_a	0.5	0.999		0.4995	0.999	

*The strength of evidence during the first two phases showed that the first treatment is Strong to Very Strong.

7. Celeration Line

A minimum of 8 data values or points in baseline is required to calculate and/or identify the location of the celeration line. Therefore, the line cannot be derived in this example. **This rule applies to all the remaining exercises in Part II.**

8. χ^2 Analysis

Phases	Below (Undesired)*	Above (Desired)**
A_1	5	5
B_1	0	9

* and **: Below or Above the Celeration Line. See Part I for further details.

$\chi^2 (n = 19) = 6.107, p < 0.05$ (Significant)

STATISTICAL ANALYSIS FOR EXAMPLE 2
(Clinical and Rehabilitation Psychology)

Data from Table C–2: Patient's anxiety levels (Social Phobia Scores)—A-B Design.

A_1 = Baseline 1, B_1 = Intervention 1

Using the statistical software packages, like SPSS, SAS, MINITAB 14, and so on, we can perform several analyses as follows.

1. Descriptive Statistics

A_1: MEAN = 16.33, MEDIAN = 16, SD = 1.527, n = 3
B_1: MEAN = 9.11, MEDIAN = 8, SD = 2.420, n = 9

Correlation Coefficients: r (A_1 and B_1) = 0.865

μ (A_1 and B_1) = 10.917

2. Analysis of Variance

(i)   For the two phases (A_1 and B_1)

Sources	SS	df	MS = SS/df	F	p	Significance
Between	117.361	1	40.111	22.764	<0.01	Highly significant
Within	51.556	10	5.1556			

3. Mann-Whitney U Test

(j)   For the first two phases (A_1 and B_1)
U = 0.00, Z = 2.49, p <0.05 (Significant)

4. *t*-test

(k)   For the first two phases (A_1 and B_1)
$t(10)$ = 4.771, p = 0.000 (Highly significant)

5. Time-Series Analysis

Phases	C	$Z = C/SE$	p-value	Significance
A_1	−0.071	−0.202	0.580	Not significant
B_1	0.840	2.839	0.002	Highly significant
A_1 and B_1	0.878	3.322	0.001	Highly significant

Where $SE = SQR\ [(n-2)/(n+1)(n-1)]$, $C = 1-[\Sigma(X_i-X_{i+1})^2/2\Sigma(X-\mu)^2]$, and $Z = C/SE$

6. Bayesian Analysis

Hypothesis: H_0: No Effect, H_a: An Effect Exists

(1) For the first two phases (A_1 and B_1)

Data	(X_i-X_{i+1})	$(X_i-X_{i+1})^2$	$(X-\mu)$	$(X-\mu)^2$	Phases
16	1	1	5.083	25.84	A_1
15	−3	9	4.083	16.67	
18	4	16	7.083	50.17	
14	2	4	3.083	9.504	B_2
12	2	4	1.083	1.173	
10	2	4	−0.917	0.84	
8	0	0	−2.917	8.51	
8	0	0	−2.917	8.51	
8	1	1	−2.917	8.51	
7	−1	1	−3.917	15.34	
8	1	1	−2.917	8.51	
7	—	—	−3.917	15.34	
SUM (Σ)		41		168.917	

Therefore, we can obtain the values of C, SE, and Z (by the formulas shown under Time-Series Analysis) as follows.

$n = 12$, SE = 0.264, C = 0.878, and Z = 3.322 ($p = 0.001$ is also called "Likelihood").

Keep repeating this process, we eventually are able to calculate Likelihood, Bayes Factor (the ratio of likelihoods), and posterior probability of each consecutive phases (See Questions 34 and 36 in Part I for further details.)

The following table shows a summary of the results of each phase.

Phases	Hypothesis	Prior Probability	Likelihood	Bayes Factor (λ)	Prior × Likelihood	Posterior Probability	
A_1B_1	H_o	0.5	0.001	0.001	0.0005	0.001	Strong to Very Strong Treatment Effect*
	H_a	0.5	0.999		0.4995	0.999	

*The strength of evidence during the first two phases showed that the first treatment is Strong to Very Strong.

7. Celeration Line

A minimum of eight data points in both phases including at least four data points in baseline is required to calculate and/or identify the location of the celeration line. Therefore, the line cannot be derived in this example. **This rule applies to all of the remaining exercises in Part II.**

8. χ^2 Analysis

Phases	Below (Undesired)*	Above (Desired)**
A_1	5	5
B_1	0	9

* and **: Below or Above the Celeration Line. See Part I for further details.

χ^2 ($n = 19$) = 6.107, p <0.05 (Significant)

SECTION D

Single Subject Designs in the Assessment of Speech and Hearing Following Cochlear Implants

Overview

Cochlear implantation has become a commonly practiced intervention to augment hearing in individuals with hearing loss. It is used in specific populations of hearing-impaired individuals, particularly in those who do not respond to more traditional acoustic amplification methods such as the use of exterior hearing aids. With cochlear implants, individuals may receive improved auditory signals and feedback. This may in turn assist individuals with speech perception, phonation, and articulation.

A typical cochlear implant (CI) involves an electrode or an array of electrodes inserted into the inner ear which may then stimulate auditory nerve fibers. The electrodes are connected to an externally attached speech processor tuned to a certain range of frequencies and amplitudes. Electrode lengths vary to reach different tonotopic regions of the cochlea: Short electrodes

can be used to reach up to about 10 millimeters into the basilar end of the cochlea. Current technology enables long electrodes to reach almost the full length of the cochlea. The individual's range of frequency loss is, to some degree, factored into decisions about electrode length and configuration. There are many other variables associated with cochlear implantation such as the type of electrode and the surgical method.

Audiologists and speech-language pathologists are critically involved with the larger clinical processes around cochlear implantation (see Proops, 2006). Most obviously, they carry out comprehensive pre- and postoperative assessments of the individual's hearing, speech, and language. Vital decisions about eligibility for CI, the target frequency range, electrode length, and so on, and about various postoperative strategies, hinge on these assessments. Many pros and cons of CI and mixed results in terms of clinical outcome are continually discussed in the research literature (see Cooper &

Craddock, 2006). The clinician plays a complex role in the multitude of auditory, speech, and language variables that are examined in exploring the effectiveness of CI. Clinical audiologists may be involved with everything from simple frequency/tone audiometric measures to measures of evoked auditory brainstem responses, pre- and post-CI or in assessing different types of CIs (see Cullington, 2003; Waltzman & Cohen, 2000). Similarly, the speech-language pathologist may assess CI effectiveness by examining speech perception abilities and language achievement in many scenarios, for example, between pre- and postimplant conditions in children (Osberger, Miyamoto, Zimmerman-Phillips, et al., 1991); between congenitally deaf children with CIs and those who receive implants after losing hearing within the first few years of life (Osberger, Todd, Berry, et al., 1991); between children wearing conventional hearing aids versus those with CIs (Miyamoto, Osberger, Robbins, et al., 1991; Tomblin, Spencer, Flock, et al., 1999); and between children who receive CIs in the prelingual ages and those who receive CIs in postlingual ages (Fryauf-Bertschy, Tyler, Kelsay et al., 1997; Tyler, Fryauf-Bertschy, Kelsay, et al., 1997); and with a range of rehabilitation scenarios with adults (see Pedley, Giles, & Hogan, 2005) Voice quality and sound production changes are often examined in individuals pre- and post-CI (Leder, Spitzer, & Kirchner, 1987) or between conditions in which the CIs are either on or off (Tye-Murray, Spencer, Bedia, and Woodworthy, 1996).

In the kinds of scenarios sampled above where there is a need to examine CI clinical outcomes, the value of single subject designs is particularly great. The large intersubject variability seen patients with CIs, especially in pediatric CI patients, makes it very difficult to achieve a large, uniform group of subjects in which the same set of variables can be studied (Higgins, McCleary, & Schulte, 1999). Assessment measures such as tone and frequency hearing thresholds; voice frequencies; vowel and consonant features; and word and language recognition will often be determined by the individual's particular pre- and postoperative conditions and by the type of implant (see above). The clinician may also need to compare changes in the patient that occur rapidly, for example, if a week after implantation, the CI is turned off for 2 days to compare hearing and speech values to earlier values.

Examples of Research Studies on Cochlear Implant Effectiveness Where Single Subject Designs Have Been Employed

A single subject design was employed by Gantz and Turner (2004) to examine speech and hearing perception in nine postlingually adult patients with high-frequency hearing loss, following CIs. The study looked at the effects of combining CI high-frequency stimulation with the patients' low-frequency hearing that, in some subjects, was assisted by a conventional hearing aid. A second question had to do with effects of different short electrodes, 6 mm and 10 mm into the basal end, inserted into the cochlea, asking whether this would preserve the acoustic low-frequency hearing and influence speech perception. Speech perception was assessed with tests of monosyllabic word and consonant recognition. Subjects were assessed preoperatively; the implant was tuned 1 month following the operation; subjects were tested at 3 months postimplantation and at various follow periods, mostly 6 to 12 months. Some subjects used the CI for less than 12 months. The subjects fitted with the 6-mm electrode showed on average a 10% improvement with consonant recognition when compared to their performance using the hearing aids only. The subjects with the 10-mm electrodes showed about a 40% gain on the task. The data on each subject also showed that with time (each successive postoperative assessment), speech recognition improved. Results pointed to the benefits of combining CI high-frequency stimulation with acoustic low-frequency hearing, and to the gains achieved with a 10-mm electrode without any effect on low-frequency hearing.

Higgins, McClearly, and Schulte (1999) used a single subject design to examine whether short-term deactivation of CIs (i.e., auditory feedback deprivation) in children would result in phonatory changes. The subjects were two prelingually deafened 6-year-old children who had been using their CIs for 2½ years, and had high speech perception and speech production skills. The subjects performed a syllable production task while intraoral air pressure, phonatory air flow, electroglottograph, fundamental frequency, and intensity measures were taken. Baseline testing was carried out over 2 days. This was followed by 3 days of experimental testing; data were collected while the subjects had their CIs turned on and when they had them turned off, on each of the 3 days. The baseline data showed the measures of phonatory behavior to vary widely in both subjects. The data from the experimental trials also varied: The subject who had better speech skills showed low intraoral air pressure and fundamental frequency scores when tested with the CI off, and this was in contrast to the subject's baseline performance. This implied that the subject had been using auditory feedback to adjust phonatory behavior. The other subject showed an increase in phonatory airflow and a small decrease in fundamental fre-

quency in the CI-off condition. As these changes did not significantly differ from the subject's baseline measurement, they could not be attributed to diminished auditory feedback. The overall mixed results suggested great complexity in how prelingually deaf children use auditory feedback, with some subjects possibly needing more time to make adjustments when feedback is diminished.

Miyamoto, Kirk, Renshaw, and Hussain (1999) employed a single subject design to evaluate the use of CIs in cases of auditory neuropathy. (Auditory neuropathy is the clinical condition of sensorineural hearing loss where otoacoustic emissions are present but the auditory evoked potential is absent; hence, the hearing loss is thought to have a central nervous system basis.) A single subject, a 4-year-old child, performed word-recognition tasks in a repeated measures design. The subject was tested on four measures of word recognition, two measures only preoperatively (due to fatigue) and all four measures at 6- and 12-month postoperative intervals. Data from matched control CI subjects (with no auditory neuropathy) were available for comparison. The only noticeable effect was that the subject's vowel recognition increased by the 12-month period. Consonant recognition declined slightly between 6 months and 12 months. Vowel and consonant recognition scores at 6 and 12 months were slightly lower than the average control scores. Word and phoneme recognition showed little or no improvement when compared to baseline measures and were far below control values. Altogether, the data showed inconclusive results with CIs used in children with auditory neuropathy and the study sounded a cautionary note.

In the three studies discussed above, single subject designs offered utility for a number of reasons. Clearly, with specific electrode configurations and surgical techniques in CIs, a large subject pool was not readily available. Testing also had to be conducted at specific pre- and postoperative intervals to necessarily monitor the few cases in question. Each study focused on a different subset of complex clinical variables and often a variable would have to be manipulated with a short course of time (e.g., turning the CI on and off in the same day). Single subject designs are therefore very practical to the clinical circumstances and logistics of CI clinical research.

Examples of Data Sets (two hypothetical cases)

We consider two scenarios, one that fits an A-B-A design and the other that fits an alternating measures design.

Example 1

A subject suffered permanent hearing loss at age 10 due to a severe, untreated inner ear infection. Hearing loss was approximately in the 2000 Hz to 7000 Hz range. Hearing aid acoustic amplification reduced this loss by a small degree, to the 3000 Hz to 7000 Hz range. The quality of the subject's voice (fundamental frequency) was affected due to lack of auditory feedback. At age 20, the subject received a CI, an electrode that stimulated hair cells in approximately the 3000 Hz to 7000 Hz region of the cochlea. Many measures were taken pre- and postoperatively. In addition to measuring the subject's fundamental frequency, a clinician used a scale of 1 to 10 to rate how closely the subject's fundamental frequency matched the normal level. One baseline (preoperative) rating was carried

out and it was very low. One month after the implant, the first postoperative rating was made, followed by four more at 1-month intervals. These ratings suggested a steady gain in voice quality over this 5-month period. At about 6-months postoperation, the subject suffered complications with the CI and it had to be removed. In the following 3 months, the subject's voice quality was again rated by the clinician. The ratings suggested a marked drop in voice quality. Table D–1 and Figure D–1 illustrate the data.

Go to Statistical Analysis for Example 1.

Example 2

A 5-year-old child suffered prelingual hearing loss with consequent impact on language learning. Speech-language assessment revealed that the subject was able to learn consonants well but had difficulty learning and recognizing vowel sounds. Comprehensive audiologic assessment identified hearing in the range of 2500 Hz and lower to be affected. The subject was implanted with a CI, a long electrode corresponding to the affected cochlear regions. Prior to the implantation, the subject's performance on vowel and consonant recognition tests were recorded in three baseline trials, 1 week apart. The tests, each scored on a scale of 1 to 8, revealed near-normal performance on consonant recognition but far lower scores for vowel recognition. The measures were then taken at 1-, 2-, and 3-month intervals postimplant, and for each of these trials, the measures were taken in alternating "on" and "off" CI conditions. In the off-conditions, performance was very similar to baseline conditions. In the on-condition, vowel recognition increased significantly and consonant recognition showed a small increase. Table D–2 and Figure D–2 illustrate the data.

Go to Statistical Analysis for Example 2.

Table D–1. Ratings of patient's voice quality (F_0) once before implantation, 4 times postimplantation, and 3 times after the implant was removed (at 1-month intervals)

Rating of Voice (F_0)	3	5	7	7	8	7	4	3	4
Trials	1	2	3	4	5	6	7	8	9

Preimplant — CI — Postimplant — CI removed at 6 months postimplant — Implant Removed

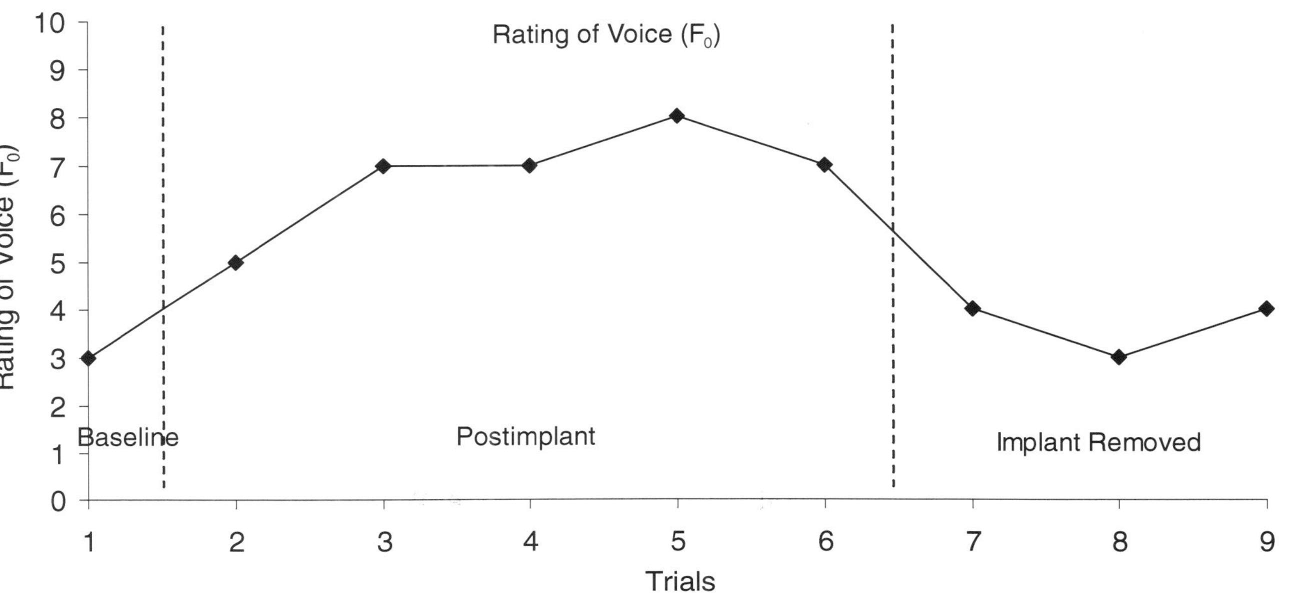

Figure D–1. Graphical illustration of ratings of patient's voice quality.

Table D–2. Patient's vowel and consonant recognition scores over 3 weeks preimplantation (baseline) and 3 weeks postimplantation during CI ON and OFF conditions

	Preimplant (weeks)				Postimplant (months)		
Vowel Recognition	2	3	4	CI ON	6	7	6
				CI OFF	3	2	3
Consonant Recognition	7	6	8	CI ON	8	7	7
				CI OFF	7	6	7
Trials	1	2	3		4	5	6

(F0)

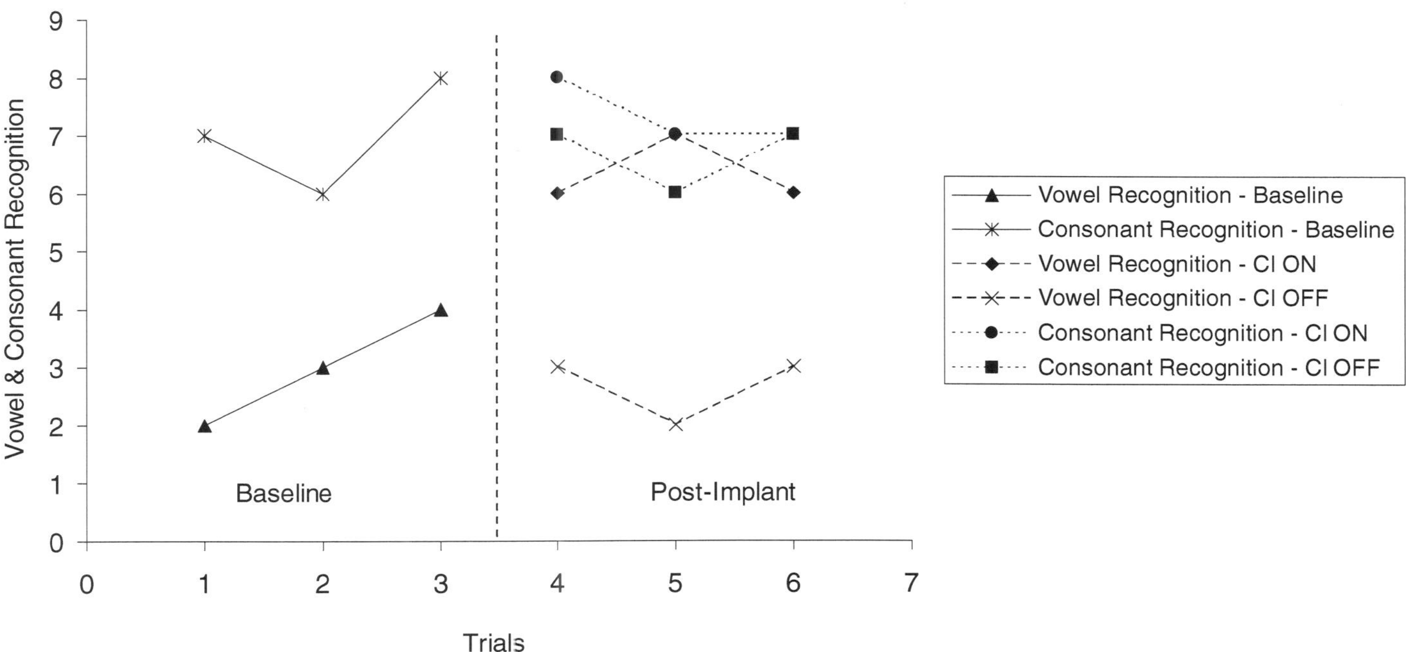

Figure D–2. Graphical illustration of patient's vowel and consonant recognition scores during preimplant and postimplant conditions.

STATISTICAL ANALYSIS FOR EXAMPLE 1
(Cochlear Implants)

Data from Table D–1: Rating of patient's voice quality (F_0) once before implantation, 4 times postimplantation, and 3 times after the implant was removed (at 1-month intervals)—A-B-A Design.

A_1 = Baseline 1, B_1 = Intervention 1, A_2 = Withdrawal

Using the statistical software packages, like SPSS, SAS, MINITAB 14, and so forth, we can perform several analyses as follows.

1. **Descriptive Statistics**

    A_1: MEAN = 3.00, MEDIAN = 3, SD = 0, $n = 1$
    B_1: MEAN = 6.80, MEDIAN = 7, SD = 1.095, $n = 5$
    A_2: MEAN = 3.66, MEDIAN = 4, SD = 0.577, $n = 3$

    Correlation Coefficients: r (A_1 and B_1) = −0.918, r (B_1 and A_2) = −0.645

    μ (A_1 and B_1) = 6.17, μ(B_1 and A_2) = 5.625

2. **Mann-Whitney U Test**

    (a) For the first two phases (A_1 and B_1)
        U = 0.00, Z = 1.46, p >0.05 (Not significant)

    (b) For the next two phases (B_1 and A_2)
        U = 0.00, Z = 2.23, p <0.05 (Significant)

3. **Time-Series Analysis**

Phases	C	$Z = C/SE$	p-value	Significance
A_1	0.000	0.000	0.500	Not significant
B_1	0.375	1.060	0.144	Not significant
A_1 and B_1	0.702	2.079	0.018	Significant
A_2	−0.500	−1.414	0.921	Not significant

Where SE = SQR $[(n-2)/(n+1)(n-1)]$, C = $1-[\Sigma(X_i-X_{i+1})^2/2\Sigma(X-\mu)^2]$, and Z = C/SE

4. Bayesian Analysis

Hypothesis: H_o: No Effect, H_a: An Effect Exists

(c) For the first two phases (A_1 and B_1)

Data	(X_i-X_{i+1})	$(X_i-X_{i+1})^2$	$(X-\mu)$	$(X-\mu)^2$	Phases
3	−2	4	−3.17	10.0489	A_1
5	−2	4	−1.17	1.3689	B_1
7	0	0	0.83	0.6889	
7	−1	1	0.83	0.6889	
8	1	1	1.83	3.3489	
7	—	—	0.83	0.6889	
SUM (Σ)		10		16.8334	

Therefore, we can obtain the values of C, SE, and Z (by the formulas shown under Time-Series Analysis) as follows.

$n = 6$, SE = 0.338, C = 0.703, and Z = 2.08 ($p = 0.018$ is also called "Likelihood").

Keep repeating this process, we eventually are able to calculate Likelihood, Bayes Factor (the ratio of likelihoods), and posterior probability of each consecutive phases (See Questions 34 and 36 in Part I for further details.)

The following table shows a summary of the results of each phase.

Phases	Hypothesis	Prior Probability	Likelihood	Bayes Factor (λ)	Prior × Likelihood	Posterior Probability	
A_1B_1	H_o	0.5	0.018	0.01833	0.009	0.018	Moderate to Strong Treatment Effect*
	H_a	0.5	0.982		0.491	0.982	
B_1A_2	H_o	0.018	0.018	0.01833	0.000324	0.000336	Moderate to Strong Withdrawal Effect**
	H_a	0.982	0.982		0.964324	0.999664	

*The strength of evidence during the first two phases showed that the first treatment is Moderate to Strong.

**The strength of evidence during the second two phases showed that the withdrawal effect is Moderate to Strong.

STATISTICAL ANALYSIS FOR EXAMPLE 2
(Cochlear Implants)

Data from Table D-2: Patient's vowel and consonant recognition scores over 3 weeks post-implantation (baseline) and 3 weeks postimplantation during CI ON and CI OFF conditions—A-B Design.

A_1 = Baseline 1, B_1 = Intervention 1

Using the statistical software packages, like SPSS, SAS, MINITAB 14, and so forth, we can perform several analyses as follows.

Vowel Recognition CI ON

1. Descriptive Statistics

A_1: MEAN = 3.00, MEDIAN = 3, SD = 1, $n = 3$
B_1: MEAN = 6.33, MEDIAN = 6, SD = 0.577, $n = 3$

Correlation Coefficients: r (A_1 and B_1) = 0.000

μ (A_1 and B_1) = 4.33

2. Analysis of Variance

(d) For the two phases (A_1 and B_1)

Sources	SS	df	MS = SS/df	F	p	Significance
Between	16.667	1	16.667	25.0	0.0075	Highly significant
Within	2.667	4	0.667			

3. Mann-Whitney U Test

(e) For the first two phases (A_1 and B_1)

U = 0.00, Z = 1.96, p <0.05 (Significant)

4. *t*-test

(f) For the first two phases (A_1 and B_1)

$t(4)$ = 5.000, p = 0.007 (Highly significant)

5. Time-Series Analysis

Phases	*C*	Z = C/SE	*p*-value	Significance
A_1	0.500	1.414	0.078	Not significant
B_1	−0.500	−1.414	0.921	Not significant
A_1 and B_1	0.793	2.346	0.009	Highly significant

Where SE = SQR $[(n-2)/(n+1)(n-1)]$, C = $1-[\Sigma(X_i-X_{i+1})^2/2\Sigma(X-\mu)^2]$, and Z = C/SE

6. Bayesian Analysis

Hypothesis: H_o: No Effect, H_a: An Effect Exists

(g) For the first two phases (A_1 and B_1)

Data	(X_i-X_{i+1})	$(X_i-X_{i+1})^2$	$(X-\mu)$	$(X-\mu)^2$	Phases
2	−1	1	−2.33	5.4289	A_1
3	−1	1	−1.33	1.7689	
4	−2	4	−0.33	0.1089	
6	−1	1	1.67	2.7889	B_1
7	1	1	2.67	7.1289	
6	—	—	1.67	2.7889	
Sum (Σ)		8		20.0134	

Therefore, we can obtain the values of C, SE, and Z (by the formulas shown under Time-Series Analysis) as follows.

$n = 6$, SE = 0.3381, C = 0.800, and Z = 2.346 ($p = 0.009$ is also called "Likelihood").

Keep repeating this process, we eventually are able to calculate Likelihood, Bayes Factor (the ratio of likelihoods), and posterior probability of each consecutive phases (See Questions 34 and 36 in Part I for further details.)

The following table shows a summary of the results of each phase.

Phases	Hypothesis	Prior Probability	Likelihood	Bayes Factor (λ)	Prior × Likelihood	Posterior Probability	
A_1B_1	H_o	0.5	0.009	0.00908	0.0045	0.009	Moderate to Strong Treatment Effect*
	H_a	0.5	0.991		0.4955	0.991	

*The strength of evidence during the first two phases showed that the first treatment is Moderate to Strong.

Vowel Recognition CI OFF

1. Descriptive Statistics

A_1: MEAN = 3.00, MEDIAN = 3, SD = 1, $n = 3$
B_1: MEAN = 2.66, MEDIAN = 3, SD = 0.577, $n = 3$

Correlation Coefficients: r (A_1 and B_1) = 0.000

μ (A_1 and B_1) = 2.83

2. Analysis of Variance

(h) For the two phases (A_1 and B_1)

Sources	SS	df	MS = SS/df	F	p	Significance
Between	0.167	1	0.167	0.25	0.6433	Not significant
Within	2.667	4	0.667			

3. Mann-Whitney U Test

(i) For the first two phases (A_1 and B_1)

U = 3.5, Z = 0.43, p >0.05 (Not significant)

4. t-test

(j) For the first two phases (A_1 and B_1)

$t(4) = 0.499$, $p = 0.643$ (Not significant)

5. Time-Series Analysis

Phases	C	$Z = C/SE$	p-value	Significance
A_1	0.500	1.414	0.078	Not significant
B_1	−0.500	−1.414	0.921	Not significant
A_1 and B_1	0.117	0.348	0.363	Not significant

Where SE = SQR $[(n-2)/(n+1)(n-1)]$, C = $1-[\Sigma(X_i-X_{i+1})^2/2\Sigma(X-\mu)^2]$, and Z = C/SE

6. Bayesian Analysis

Hypothesis: H_o: No Effect, H_a: An Effect Exists

(k) For the first two phases (A_1 and B_1)

Data	(X_i-X_{i+1})	$(X_i-X_{i+1})^2$	$(X-\mu)$	$(X-\mu)^2$	Phases
2	−1	1	−0.83	0.6889	A_1
3	−1	1	0.17	0.0289	
4	1	1	1.17	1.3689	
3	1	1	0.17	0.0289	B_1
2	−1	1	−0.83	0.6889	
3	—	—	0.17	0.0289	
Sum (Σ)		5		2.8334	

Therefore, we can obtain the values of C, SE, and Z (by the formulas shown under Time-Series Analysis) as follows.

$n = 6$, SE = 0.3381, C = 0.1177, and Z = 0.348 (p = 0.363 is also called "Likelihood").

Keep repeating this process, we eventually are able to calculate Likelihood, Bayes Factor (the ratio of likelihoods), and posterior probability of each consecutive phases (See Questions 34 and 36 in Part I for further details.)

The following table shows a summary of the results of each phase.

Phases	Hypothesis	Prior Probability	Likelihood	Bayes Factor (λ)	Prior × Likelihood	Posterior Probability	
A_1B_1	H_o	0.5	0.363	0.57	0.1815	0.363	Weak Treatment Effect*
	H_a	0.5	0.637		0.3185	0.637	

*The strength of evidence during the first two phases showed that the first treatment is Weak.

Consonant Recognition CI ON

1. Descriptive Statistics

A_1: MEAN = 7.00, MEDIAN = 7, SD = 1, $n = 3$
B_1: MEAN = 7.33, MEDIAN = 7, SD = 0.577, $n = 3$

Correlation Coefficients: r (A_1 and B_1) = 0.000

μ (A_1 and B_1) = 7.17

2. Analysis of Variance

(1)   For the two phases (A_1 and B_1)

Sources	SS	df	MS = SS/df	*F*	*p*	Significance
Between	0.167	1	0.167	0.25	0.6433	Not significant
Within	2.667	4	0.667			

3. Mann-Whitney U Test

(m) For the first two phases (A_1 and B_1)
   U = 3.5, Z = 0.43, p >0.05 (Not significant)

4. *t*-test

(n) For the first two phases (A_1 and B_1)
   $t(4) = 0.499$, $p = 0.643$ (Not significant)

5. Time-Series Analysis

Phases	*C*	Z = C/SE	*p*-value	Significance
A_1	−0.250	−0.707	0.760	Not significant
B_1	0.250	0.707	0.239	Not significant
A_1 and B_1	−0.058	−0.174	0.569	Not significant

Where SE = SQR $[(n-2)/(n+1)(n-1)]$, C = $1-[\Sigma(X_i-X_{i+1})^2/2\Sigma(X-\mu)^2]$, and Z = C/SE

6. Bayesian Analysis

Hypothesis: H_o: No Effect, H_a: An Effect Exists

For the first two phases (A_1 and B_1)

Data	(X_i-X_{i+1})	$(X_i-X_{i+1})^2$	$(X-\mu)$	$(X-\mu)^2$	Phases
7	1	1	0.17	0.0289	A_1
6	−2	4	−1.17	1.3689	
8	0	0	0.83	0.6889	
8	1	1	0.83	0.6889	B_1
7	0	0	−0.17	0.0289	
7	—	—	−0.17	0.0289	
Sum (Σ)		6		2.8334	

Therefore, we can obtain the values of C, SE, and Z (by the formulas shown under Time-Series Analysis) as follows.

$n = 6$, SE $= 0.3381$, C $= -0.0588$, and Z $= -0.174$ ($p = 0.569$ is also called "Likelihood").

Keep repeating this process, we eventually are able to calculate Likelihood, Bayes Factor (the ratio of likelihoods), and posterior probability of each consecutive phases (See Questions 34 and 36 in Part I for further details.)

The following table shows a summary of the results of each phase.

Phases	Hypothesis	Prior Probability	Likelihood	Bayes Factor (λ)	Prior × Likelihood	Posterior Probability	
A_1B_1	H_o	0.5	0.569	1.32	0.2845	0.569	Weak Treatment Effect*
	H_a	0.5	0.431		0.2155	0.431	

*The strength of evidence during the first two phases showed that the first treatment is Weak.

Consonant Recognition CI OFF

1. Descriptive Statistics

A_1: MEAN = 7.00, MEDIAN = 7, SD = 1, $n = 3$
B_1: MEAN = 6.66, MEDIAN = 7, SD = 0.577, $n = 3$

Correlation Coefficients: r (A_1 and B_1) = 0.866

μ (A_1 and B_1) = 6.83

2. Analysis of Variance

(p) For the two phases (A_1 and B_1)

Sources	SS	df	MS = SS/df	*F*	*p*	Significance
Between	0.167	1	0.167	0.25	0.6433	Not significant
Within	2.667	4	0.667			

3. Mann-Whitney U Test

(q) For the first two phases (A_1 and B_1)
$U = 3.5$, $Z = 0.43$, $p > 0.05$ (Not significant)

4. *t*-test

(r) For the first two phases (A_1 and B_1)
$t(4) = 0.499$, $p = 0.643$ (Not significant)

5. Time-Series Analysis

Phases	*C*	Z = C/SE	*p*-value	Significance
A_1	−0.250	−0.707	0.760	Not significant
B_1	−0.500	−1.414	0.921	Not significant
A_1 and B_1	−0.411	−1.218	0.888	Not significant

Where SE = SQR $[(n-2)/(n+1)(n-1)]$, C = $1 - [\Sigma(X_i - X_{i+1})^2 / 2\Sigma(X - \mu)^2]$, and Z = C/SE

6. Bayesian Analysis

Hypothesis: H_o: No Effect, H_a: An Effect Exists

(s) For the first two phases (A_1 and B_1)

Data	(X_i-X_{i+1})	$(X_i-X_{i+1})^2$	$(X-\mu)$	$(X-\mu)^2$	Phases
7	1	1	0.17	0.0289	A_1
6	−2	4	−0.83	0.6889	
8	1	1	1.17	1.3689	
7	1	1	0.17	0.0289	B_1
6	−1	1	−0.83	0.6889	
7	—	—	0.17	0.0289	
Sum (Σ)		8		2.8334	

Therefore, we can obtain the values of C, SE, and Z (by the formulas shown under Time-Series Analysis) as follows.

$N = 6$, $SE = 0.3381$, $C = −0.412$, and $Z = −1.219$ ($p = 0.888$ is also called "Likelihood").

Keep repeating this process, we eventually are able to calculate Likelihood, Bayes Factor (the ratio of likelihoods), and posterior probability of each consecutive phases (See Questions 34 and 36 in Part I for further details.)

The following table shows a summary of the results of each phase.

Phases	Hypothesis	Prior Probability	Likelihood	Bayes Factor (λ)	Prior × Likelihood	Posterior Probability	
A_1B_1	H_o	0.5	0.888	7.93	0.444	0.888	Very Weak Treatment Effect*
	H_a	0.5	0.112		0.056	0.112	

*The strength of evidence during the first two phases showed that the first treatment is Very Weak.

Vowel Recognition CI ON Versus CI OFF (Inferential Approach)

1. Descriptive Statistics

CI ON: MEAN = 4.66, MEDIAN = 5, SD = 1.966, $n = 6$
CI OFF: MEAN = 2.83, MEDIAN = 3, SD = 0.752, $n = 6$

Correlation Coefficients: r (A_1 and B_1) = −0.045

μ (A_1 and B_1) = 3.75

2. Autocorrelation Coefficients- Product-Moment lag-1: CI ON and CI OFF

CI ON: $r = 0.851$, $p = 0.06741$ (Not significant)
CI OFF: $r = 0.00$, $p = 1.0$ (Not significant)

3. Analysis of Variance: CI ON versus CI OFF

Sources	SS	df	MS = SS/df	F	p	Significance
Between	10.083	1	10.083	4.549	0.0587	Not significant
Within	22.167	10	2.217			

4. Mann-Whitney U Test

U = 8.0, Z = 1.60, p >0.05 (Not significant)

5. *t*-test

$t(10) = 2.132$, $p = 0.058$ (Not significant)

6. Time-Series Analysis

Phases	C	Z = C/SE	p-value	Significance
CI ON	0.793	2.346	0.009	Highly significant
CI OFF	0.117	0.348	0.363	Not significant
ON and OFF	0.550	2.081	0.018	Significant

Where SE = SQR $[(n-2)/(n+1)(n-1)]$, C = $1-[\Sigma(X_i-X_{i+1})^2/2\Sigma(X-\mu)^2]$, and Z = C/SE

Consonant Recognition CI ON Versus CI OFF (Inferential Approach)

1. Descriptive Statistics

CI ON: MEAN = 7.16, MEDIAN = 7, SD = 0.752, $n = 6$
CI OFF: MEAN = 6.83, MEDIAN = 7, SD = 0.752, $n = 6$

Correlation Coefficients: r (A_1 and B_1) = 0.764

μ (A_1 and B_1) = 7.00

2. Autocorrelation Coefficients- Product-Moment lag-1: CI ON and CI OFF

CI ON: r = -0.071, p = 0.90913 (Not significant)
CI OFF: r = −0.428, p = 0.47153 (Not significant)

3. Analysis of Variance: CI ON versus CI OFF

(t)   For the two phases (A_1 and B_1)

Sources	SS	df	MS = SS/df	F	p	Significance
Between	0.333	1	0.333	0.588	0.4608	Not significant
Within	5.667	10	0.567			

4. Mann-Whitney U Test

U = 13.5, Z = 0.72, p >0.05 (Not significant)

5. *t*-test

$t(10)$ = 0.766, p = 0.460 (Not significant)

6. Time-Series Analysis

Phases	C	Z = C/SE	p-value	Significance
CI ON	−0.058	−0.174	0.569	Not significant
CI OFF	−0.411	−1.218	0.888	Not significant
ON and OFF	−0.166	−0.630	0.735	Not significant

Where SE = SQR $[(n−2)/(n+1)(n−1)]$, C = $1−[\Sigma(X_i−X_{i+1})^2/2\Sigma(X−\mu)^2]$, and Z = C/SE

SECTION E

Single Subject Designs in Training Interventions for Children with Autism

Overview

Clinicians in communication disorders often play central roles in assessment and intervention with individuals who are developmentally delayed or who have specific neurodevelopmental disorders. Deficits in verbal and nonverbal communication are among the most profound across the range of neurodevelopmental disorders (Baron-Cohen, Tager-Flusberg, & Cohen, 2000). These disorders have multiple levels of complexity. A single type of neurodevelopmental disorder, for example, autism, has varying patterns of behavioral manifestations, varying rates of progression, and numerous etiologic factors. Hence, enormous challenges arise not only in terms of the neurocognitive understanding of such disorders but also therapeutic interventions.

Autism is an especially good case in point. In children with autism, there is often an instability in the cognitive profile in the very early years of life and the condition can be difficult to diagnose during this time (Bernabei & Camaioni, 2001). New evaluation and intervention methods steadily evolve as the understanding of the disorder evolves (see Drew, Baird, Baron-Cohen, et al., 2002; Waitling, Deitz, Kanny, & McLaughlin, 1999). Behavioral and cognitive features of autism have been extensively documented (see Frith & Hill, 2004) and within this larger set of features, distinct forms of communication impairments have been well described (Charman, Swettenham, Baron-Cohen et al., 1997; Charman, Baron-Cohen, Swettenham, et al., 2003; Mundy, Sigman, Ungerer & Sherman, 1986). Social-cognitive-communicative impairments have been finely delineated in terms of impairments in sensory integration, joint attention, goal detection, social gaze, imitation and spontaneous play, and affective and empathic responses. Such features can be measured, for example, by timing the duration of a subject's lack of social acknowledgment; counting the number of eye contacts within a certain time period; recording the frequency of initiated interactions, gestures, and imitative behavior, the extent of interaction in play, and so on. Formal measures of these features are more often carried out in clinical research studies of autism (see Charman et al., 2003; Wimpory, Chadwick, & Nash, 1995). In more typical, everyday clinical practice, intervention with children with autism most often involves a one-to-one format, and clinicians tend to rely heavily on nonstandardized methods and observed behavior (Watling et al., 1999).

Because there is such variability in terms of therapeutic gains among subjects with autism, research methods that employ group designs that scale scores, can blur any positive results gained by some subjects (Ottenbacher, 1986). Single subject designs offer an alternative and can substantially aid a clinician with assessment and therapeutic intervention in autism. In addition to observed behavior and screening tools, the clinician can apply a single case design to profile a pattern of features in a subject. As therapy targets one or more features, the efficacy of the intervention can also be gauged using a single case design. In view of how varied the cognitive-behavioral profile across subjects can be and how a single subject's profile of features can change, the single subject design offers the clinician a means to manage an otherwise complex picture.

Examples of Training Interventions in Autism Where Single Subject Designs Have Been Employed

Case-Smith and Bryan (1999) used an A-B design to assess the effects of sensory integration on five preschool children with autism, in a preschool intervention program. Over a 3-week baseline period, three operationally defined target features, nonengagement, goal directed play, and interaction were measured through video recordings of the subjects' play behavior during free time at school. Intervention began on week 4 and involved 10 weeks of one-to-one counseling sessions with each child and consultation with teachers. Helping the subjects cope with sensory integration and helping the parents understand the subjects' sensory needs were the goals of the intervention. It involved, for example, tailoring the environment to the subjects' sensory needs; helping the subjects deal with multiple sensory input, and so on. When subjects' behavior was compared between the baseline and intervention phases, three subjects showed an increase in goal-directed play and four subjects showed a decrease in nonengaged behaviors, during intervention. Changes in frequency of interaction were minimal. The authors attributed the improvements in the intervention phase to improvement in a few areas of sensory integration.

An A-B-C design was employed by Wimpory, Chadwick, and Nash (1995) in evaluating the effect of musical interaction therapy (MIT) on a single subject. The subject was a 3-year and 3-month-old girl with severe autism. She was noncommunicative. The authors argued that music interaction therapy had a unique potential. Live music synchronized in tone, beat, rhythm, and so forth, to the child's interactions with an adult, could help cue the child to contingencies and dynamics. In this way, the child would be aided in dyadic communication, for example, by cues to anticipate the actions of the interacting partner. Five target features were measured: Social acknowledgement, eye contact, interactive involvement, initiated changes to interaction, and spontaneous play. Baseline data were collected during six home visits over 4 months. Intervention involved 20-minute MIT sessions twice a week over 7 months. It involved a musician playing a harp and matching in tone and timing the interaction between the child and her mother in game playing, vocalizing, rhyme activity, and so forth. Seven measures of the target features were made during the 7-month intervention phase. This was followed by 5 months of unmonitored MIT. Follow-up was made 20 months later. Three features, social acknowledgment, eye contact, and interactive involvement, showed improved scores after MIT was introduced. The other two features showed increased scores only in the latter parts of the intervention phase. These results were as predicted by the authors based on developmental trend lines inferred through the baseline scores. At the 20-month follow-up, the subject had maintained the improved performed. The authors suggested that the data provided preliminary evidence of the positive effects of MIT in facilitating interaction in subjects with autism.

Clinical studies of autism like those described above often have to focus on numbers of occurrences or initiations of a behavior, duration of a behavior or response, and so forth, and this has to be done under difficult circumstances—with individuals who are not well responsive or compliant. In addition, each individual's behavior is unique as is the developmental pattern of the behavior. In such conditions, the value of single subject designs is immense. Specifically targeted features can be compared within a subject across different phases of a study, and this fits very well with common therapeutic interventions in autism.

Examples of Data Sets (two hypothetical cases)

We consider two scenarios, one that fits an A-B design and the other that fits an A-B-C design, a special case of the A-B-A design. In the A-B-C design (as applied by Case-Smith

& Bryan, 1999), follow-up is separated from the intervention phase by a long time period.

Example 1

At 9 months, a child manifests features of autism. A team of clinicians decide to begin monitoring the pattern of development of certain behavioral features of the child. For purposes of establishing a baseline of behavioral features of interest, a home video monitoring program is implemented. Beginning in the 13th month of age, the child's interaction with her parents is monitored during hour-long play sessions, once a day, 5 days a week, for 6 months. Of interest is the frequency of behavioral features that fall into the subsets of physical gestures, verbal communication, and action-play schemes. After 6 months, the data are analyzed. Scores are averaged into one score a month for each of the three features. Occurrences of physical gestures and action-play schemes appear minimal whereas verbal language appears as slightly above minimal occurrence. In the 7th month, a clinician trained in facilitating interaction between an autistic child and parents, joins the daily play sessions. The clinician initiates an intervention program designed to facilitate physical gestures, verbal communication, and action-play schemes between the parent and child. The clinician applies these techniques steadily and consistently during play sessions over a period of 3 months. Analysis of the video recording during the intervention phase shows that physical gestures and action-play schemes rise sharply above baseline levels whereas verbal language rises only a small degree above baseline. The data give the clinical team a view of the developmental trajectory of the behavioral features and some indication of which features respond better to facilitative interaction. With this data, clinicians can fine tune the intervention for the next course of treatment. Table E-1 and Figure E-1 illustrate the data.

Go to Statistical Analysis for Example 1.

Example 2

Three children, all boys around 4½ years of age, had been diagnosed with autism around the age of 2 years. All earlier reports indicated that they were socially withdrawn, showed little eye contact, and lacked spontaneous play. The children have been sent to a new school where a clinician is required to treat them as a group in a school-based program. The clinician first spends 3 months recording baseline data. She engages the boys in group play for an hour per day while her assistant captures the activity on video. Frequency of eye contacts per minute, number of actions per minute,

Table E–1. Monthly averages of the daily frequencies of occurrence of target behaviors of a single subject during baseline and intervention

Physical Gestures	3	2	3	4	3	2	5	6	7
Verbal Communication	4	5	4	3	4	4	4	5	4
Action-Play Schemes	3	3	2	3	2	2	5	6	6

Months	1	2	3	4	5	6	7	8	9
	Baseline						Facilitative Intervention		

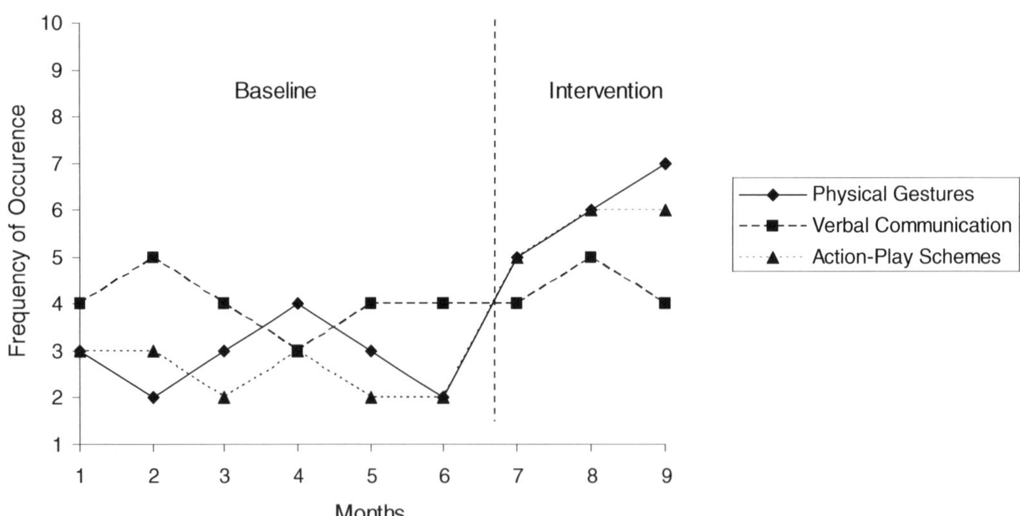

Figure E–1. Graphical illustration of monthly averages of the daily frequencies of occurrence of target behaviors of a single subject during baseline and intervention.

and number of vocalizations per minute are recorded. Each of these behaviors is depressed. The clinician decides on a course of intervention that is akin to a sensory integration model. It involves playing games with the boys while using gestures and sounds to indicate to them when to initiate or hold a behavior. Assistants are brought in. The game involves lots of little toys and balls that have to be passed, shared, and played with, at certain moments as cued by the clinician's team. Cues are in the form of gestures and drum sounds. Both forms of cues are varied to match moments of anticipation, urgency, stop-go sequences, and so forth. The intervention is made during hour-long daily sessions, over 3 months. Data recorded during intervention show a marked improvement in all measures when compared to baseline, in two of the three boys. The third boy shows minimal improvement. The school then has a 3-month long summer break. When school resumes, the boys are given a month-long follow-up. The results remain almost the same as the results from the intervention phase. The data help the clinician determine how the treatment should be continued and systematized for two of the boys and how one of the boys should be channeled into a different form of treatment. Table E–2 and Figures E–2, E–3, and E–4 illustrate the data.

Go to Statistical Analysis for Example 2.

Table E–2. Monthly averages of the daily frequencies of occurrence of target behaviors of each of three single subjects during baseline, intervention, and follow-up

		1	2	3	4	5	6	7–9	10
Subject 1	Eye Contact	2	1	4	4	6	6		5
	Actions	3	3	4	5	4	6		6
	Vocalization	3	3	2	5	5	7		6
Subject 2	Eye Contact	3	2	3	5	5	5		4
	Actions	2	4	4	6	4	5		5
	Vocalization	3	5	2	4	5	6		5
Subject 3	Eye Contact	2	1	2	2	2	4		3
	Actions	2	2	3	4	2	3		4
	Vocalization	1	2	1	2	3	2		3
	Months	1	2	3	4	5	6	7–9	10
			Baseline		Intervention (Sensory Integration)			Break	Follow-Up

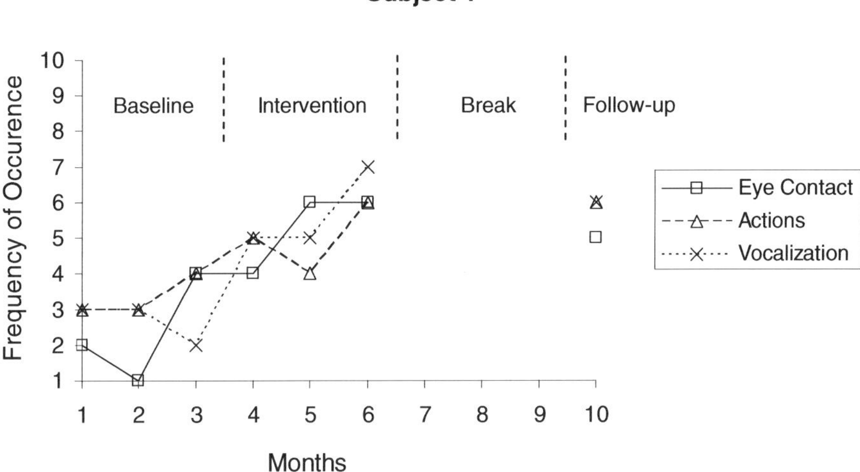

Figures E–2 to E–4. Graphical illustration of monthly averages of the daily frequencies of occurrence of target behaviors of each of three single subjects during baseline, intervention, and follow-up.

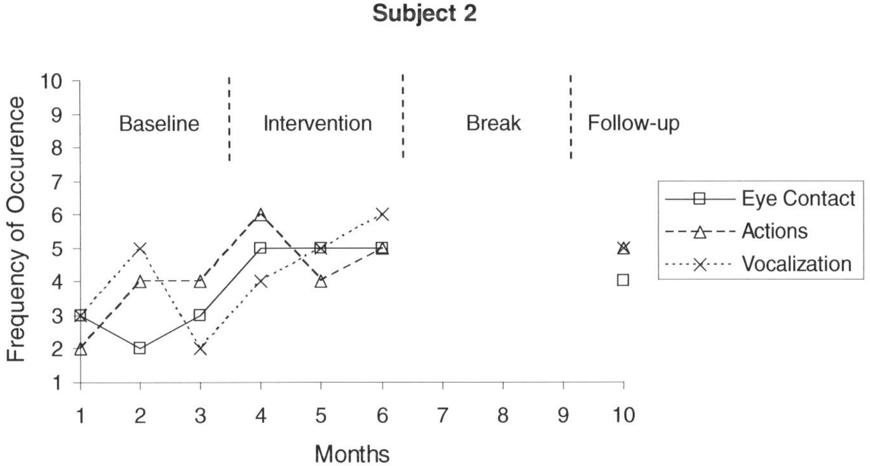

Figure E–3.

Subject 3

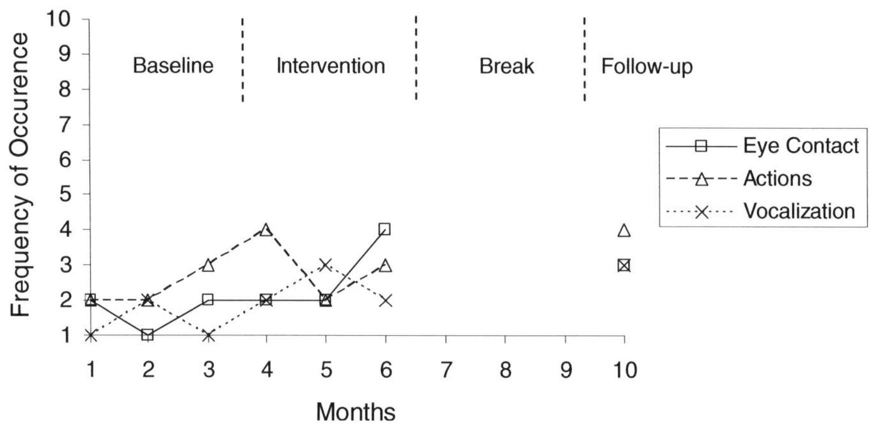

Figure E–4.

STATISTICAL ANALYSIS FOR EXAMPLE 1
(Treatment of Autism)

Data from Table E–1: Monthly averages of the daily frequencies of occurrence of target behaviors of a single subject—A-B Design.

A_1 = Baseline 1, B_1 = Intervention 1

Using the statistical software packages, like SPSS, SAS, MINITAB 14, and so forth, we can perform several analyses as follows.

Physical Gestures

1. **Descriptive Statistics**
   A_1: MEAN = 2.83, MEDIAN = 3, SD = 0.752, $n = 6$
   B_1: MEAN = 6.00, MEDIAN = 6, SD = 1, $n = 3$

   Correlation Coefficients: r (A_1 and B_1) = −0.238

   μ (A_1 and B_1) = 3.89

2. **Analysis of Variance**

Source	SS	df	MS	F	p-value
Between	20.056	1	20.056	29.046	0.0010
Within	4.833	7	0.69		Highly Significant

3. **Mann-Whitney U Test**

   For the first two phases (A_1 and B_1)
   U = 0.0, Z = 2.32, p <0.05 (Significant)

4. ***t*-test**

   $t(7) = 5.389$, $p = 0.001$ (Highly significant)

5. **Time-Series Analysis**

Phases	C	$Z = C/SE$	p-value	Significance
A_1	0.117	0.348	0.363	Not significant
B_1	0.500	1.414	0.078	Not significant
A_1 and B_1	0.678	2.293	0.011	Significant

Where SE = SQR $[(n-2)/(n+1)(n-1)]$, C = $1-[\Sigma(X_i-X_i+_1)^2/2\Sigma(X-\mu)^2]$, and Z = C/SE

6. Bayesian Analysis

Hypothesis: H_o: No Effect, H_a: An Effect Exists

For the first two phases (A_1 and B_1)

Data	$(X_i - X_{i+1})$	$(X_i - X_{i+1})^2$	$(X - \mu)$	$(X - \mu)^2$	Phases
3	1	1	−0.89	0.7921	A_1
2	−1	1	−1.89	3.5721	
3	−1	1	−0.89	0.7921	
4	1	1	0.11	0.0121	
3	1	1	−0.89	0.7921	
2	−3	9	−1.89	3.5721	
5	−1	1	1.11	1.2321	B_1
6	−1	1	2.11	4.4521	
7	—	—	3.11	9.6721	
SUM (Σ)		16		24.8889	

Therefore, we can obtain the values of C, SE, and Z (by the formulas shown under Time-Series Analysis) as follows.

$n = 9$, SE = 0.296, C = 0.6786, and Z = 2.293 (p =0.0110 is also called "Likelihood").

Keep repeating this process, we eventually are able to calculate Likelihood, Bayes Factor (the ratio of likelihoods), and posterior probability of each consecutive phases (See Questions 34 and 36 in Part I for further details.)

The following table shows a summary of the results of each phase.

Phases	Hypothesis	Prior Probability	Likelihood	Bayes Factor (λ)	Prior × Likelihood	Posterior Probability	
A_1B_1	H_o	0.5	0.0110	0.0111	0.0055	0.0110	Moderate to Strong Treatment Effect*
	H_a	0.5	0.9890	0.4945	0.9890		

*The strength of evidence during the first two phases showed that the first treatment is Moderate to Strong.

Verbal Communication

1. Descriptive Statistics

A_1: MEAN = 4.00, MEDIAN = 4, SD = 0.632, $n = 6$
B_1: MEAN = 4.33, MEDIAN = 4, SD = 0.577, $n = 3$

Correlation Coefficients: r (A_1 and B_1) = 0.658

μ (A_1 and B_1) = 4.11

2. Analysis of Variance

Source	SS	df	MS	*F*	*p*-value
Between	0.222	1	0.222	0.583	0.47
Within	2.667	7	0.381		Not Significant

3. Mann-Whitney U Test

For the first two phases (A_1 and B_1)
U = 6.5, Z = 0.64, p >0.05 (Not significant)

4. *t*-test

$t(7) = 0.763$, $p = 0.469$ (Not significant)

5. Time-Series Analysis

Phases	*C*	*Z* = C/SE	*p*-value	Significance
A_1	0.000	0.000	0.500	Not significant
B_1	−0.500	−1.414	0.921	Not significant
A_1 and B_1	−0.038	−0.130	0.551	Not significant

Where SE = SQR $[(n-2)/(n+1)(n-1)]$, C = $1-[\Sigma(X_i-X_i+_1)^2/2\Sigma(X-\mu)^2]$, and Z = C/SE

6. Bayesian Analysis

Hypothesis: H_o: No Effect, H_a: An Effect Exists

For the first two phases (A_1 and B_1)

Data	(X_i-X_{i+1})	$(X_i-X_{i+1})^2$	$(X-\mu)$	$(X-\mu)^2$	Phases
4	−1	1	−0.11	0.0121	A_1
5	1	1	0.89	0.7921	
4	1	1	−0.11	0.0121	
3	−1	1	−1.11	1.2321	
4	0	0	−0.11	0.0121	
4	0	0	−0.11	0.0121	
4	−1	1	−0.11	0.0121	B_1
5	1	1	0.89	0.7921	
4	—	—	−0.11	0.0121	
SUM (Σ)		6		2.8889	

Therefore, we can obtain the values of C, SE, and Z (by the formulas shown under Time-Series Analysis) as follows.

$n = 9$, SE $= 0.296$, C $= -0.03846$, and Z $= -0.13$ ($p = 0.5517$ is also called "Likelihood").

Keep repeating this process, we will eventually be able to calculate Likelihood, Bayes Factor (the ratio of likelihoods), and posterior probability of each consecutive phases (See Questions 34 and 36 in Part I for further details.)

The following table shows a summary of the results of each phase.

Phases	Hypothesis	Prior Probability	Likelihood	Bayes Factor (λ)	Prior × Likelihood	Posterior Probability	
A_1B_1	H_o	0.5	0.5517	1.23	0.27585	0.5517	Very Weak Treatment Effect*
	H_a	0.5	0.4483		0.22415	0.4483	

*The strength of evidence during the first two phases showed that the first treatment is Very Weak.

Action Play Schemes

1. Descriptive Statistics

A_1: MEAN = 2.50, MEDIAN = 2.50, SD = 0.547, n = 6
B_1: MEAN = 5.66, MEDIAN = 6, SD = 0.577, n = 3

Correlation Coefficients: r (A_1 and B_1) = 0.292

μ (A_1 and B_1) = 3.56

2. Analysis of Variance

Source	SS	df	MS	*F*	*p*-value
Between	20.056	1	20.056	64.795	<0.001
Within	2.167	7	0.31		Highly Significant

3. Mann-Whitney U Test

For the first two phases (A_1 and B_1)
U = 0.0, Z = 2.32, *p* <0.05 (Significant)

4. *t*-test

$t(7) = 8.049$, $p = 0.000$ (Highly significant)

5. Time-Series Analysis

Phases	*C*	*Z* = C/SE	*p*-value	Significance
A_1	0.000	0.000	0.500	Not significant
B_1	0.250	0.707	0.239	Not significant
A_1 and B_1	0.707	2.391	0.008	Highly significant

Where SE = SQR $[(n-2)/(n+1)(n-1)]$, C = $1-[\Sigma(X_i-X_i+_1)^2/2\Sigma(X-\mu)^2]$, and Z = C/SE

6. Bayesian Analysis

Hypothesis: H_o: No Effect, H_a: An Effect Exists

For the first two phases (A_1 and B_1)

Data	$(X_i - X_{i+1})$	$(X_i - X_{i+1})^2$	$(X - \mu)$	$(X - \mu)^2$	Phases
3	0	0	−0.56	0.3136	A_1
3	1	1	−0.56	0.3136	
2	−1	1	−1.56	2.4336	
3	1	1	−0.56	0.3136	
2	0	0	−1.56	2.4336	
2	−3	9	−1.56	2.4336	
5	−1	1	1.44	2.0736	B_1
6	0	0	2.44	5.9536	
6	—	—	2.44	5.9536	
SUM (Σ)		13		22.2224	

Therefore, we can obtain the values of C, SE, and Z (by the formulas shown under Time-Series Analysis) as follows.

$N = 9$, $SE = 0.296$, $C = 0.7075$, and $Z = 2.39$ ($p = 0.0084$ is also called "Likelihood").

Keep repeating this process, we eventually are able to calculate Likelihood, Bayes Factor (the ratio of likelihoods), and posterior probability of each consecutive phases (See Questions 34 and 36 in Part I for further details.)

The following table shows a summary of the results of each phase.

Phases	Hypothesis	Prior Probability	Likelihood	Bayes Factor (λ)	Prior × Likelihood	Posterior Probability	
A_1B_1	H_o	0.5	0.0084	0.00847	0.0042	0.0084	Moderate to Strong Treatment Effect*
	H_a	0.5	0.9916		0.4958	0.9916	

*The strength of evidence during the first two phases showed that the first treatment is Moderate to Strong.

STATISTICAL ANALYSIS FOR EXAMPLE 2
(Treatment of Autism)

Data from Table E–2: Monthly averages of the daily frequencies of occurrence of target behaviors of three single subjects—A-B-A Design.

A_1 = Baseline 1, B_1 = Intervention 1, A_2 = Withdrawal

Using the statistical software packages, like SPSS, SAS, MINITAB 14, and so forth, we can perform several analyses as follows.

Subject 1: Eye Contact

1. Descriptive Statistics

A_1: MEAN = 2.33, MEDIAN = 2, SD = 1.527, $n = 3$
B_1: MEAN = 5.33, MEDIAN = 6, SD = 1.154, $n = 3$
A_2: MEAN = 5.00, MEDIAN = 5, SD = 0.000, $n = 1$

Correlation Coefficients: r (A_1 and B_1) = 0.188, r (B_1 and A_2) = −1.000

μ (A_1 and B_1) = 3.83, μ(B_1 and A_2) = 5.25

2. Mann-Whitney U Test

(a) For the first two phases (A_1 and B_1)

U = 0.5, Z = 1.74, p >0.05 (Not significant)

(b) For the next two phases (B_1 and A_2)

U = 1.0, Z = 0.44, p >0.05 (Not significant)

3. Time-Series Analysis

Phases	C	$Z = C/SE$	p-**value**	**Significance**
A_1	−0.071	−0.202	0.580	Not significant
B_1	0.249	0.707	0.239	Not significant
A_1 and B_1	0.690	2.04	0.021	Significant
A_2	0.000	0.000	0.500	Not significant

Where SE = SQR $[(n-2)/(n+1)(n-1)]$, C = $1-[\Sigma(X_i-X_i+_1)^2/2\Sigma(X-\mu)^2]$, and Z = C/SE

4. Bayesian Analysis

Hypothesis: H_0: No Effect, H_a: An Effect Exists

(c) For the first two phases (A_1 and B_1)

Data	$(X_i - X_{i+1})$	$(X_i - X_{i+1})^2$	$(X - \mu)$	$(X - \mu)^2$	Phases
2	1	1	−1.286	1.6538	A_1
1	−3	9	−2.286	5.2258	
4	0	0	0.714	0.5098	
4	−2	4	0.714	0.5098	B_1
6	0	0	2.714	7.3658	
6	—	—	2.714	7.3658	
SUM (Σ)		14		22.6308	

Therefore, we can obtain the values of C, SE, and Z (by the formulas shown under Time-Series Analysis) as follows.

$n = 6$, SE = 0.338, C = 0.690, and Z = 2.04 ($p = 0.0207$ is also called "Likelihood").

Keep repeating this process, we eventually are able to calculate Likelihood, Bayes Factor (the ratio of likelihoods), and posterior probability of each consecutive phases (See Questions 34 and 36 in Part I for further details.)

The following table shows a summary of the results of each phase.

Phases	Hypothesis	Prior Probability	Likelihood	Bayes Factor (λ)	Prior × Likelihood	Posterior Probability	
$A_1 B_1$	H_0	0.5	0.0207	0.021	0.01035	0.0207	Moderate to Strong Treatment Effect*
	H_a	0.5	0.9793		0.48965	0.9793	
$B_1 A_2$	H_0	0.0207	0.3936	0.649	0.00815	0.0135	Weak Withdrawal Effect**
	H_a	0.9793	0.6064		0.59385	0.9865	

*The strength of evidence during the first two phases showed that the first treatment is Moderate to Strong.

**The strength of evidence during the second two phases showed that the withdrawal effect is Weak.

Subject 1: Actions

1. Descriptive Statistics

A_1: MEAN = 3.33, MEDIAN = 3, SD = 0.577, $n = 3$
B_1: MEAN = 5.00, MEDIAN = 5, SD = 1, $n = 3$
A_2: MEAN = 6.00, MEDIAN = 6, SD = 0, $n = 1$

Correlation Coefficients: r (A_1 and B_1) = 0.866, r (B_1 and A_2) = 0.000

μ (A_1 and B_1) = 4.17, μ(B_1 and A_2) = 5.25

2. Mann-Whitney U Test

(d) For the first two phases (A_1 and B_1)
  U = 0.5, Z = 1.74, p >0.05 (Not significant)

(e) For the next two phases (B_1 and A_2)
  U = 0.5, Z = 0.89, p >0.05 (Not significant)

3. Time-Series Analysis

Phases	C	Z = C/SE	p-value	Significance
A_1	0.249	0.707	0.239	Not significant
B_1	−0.250	−0.707	0.760	Not significant
A_1 and B_1	0.487	1.442	0.074	Not significant
A_2	0.000	0.000	0.500	Not significant

Where SE = SQR $[(n-2)/(n+1)(n-1)]$, C = $1-[\Sigma(X_i-X_i+_1)^2/2\Sigma(X-\mu)^2]$, and Z = C/SE

4. Bayesian Analysis

Hypothesis: H_o: No Effect, H_a: An Effect Exists

(f) For the first two phases (A_1 and B_1)

Data	(X_i-X_{i+1})	$(X_i-X_{i+1})^2$	$(X-\mu)$	$(X-\mu)^2$	Phases
3	0	0	−1.17	1.3689	A_1
3	−1	1	−1.17	1.3689	
4	−1	1	−0.17	0.0289	
5	1	1	0.83	0.6889	B_1
4	−2	4	−0.17	0.0289	
6	—	—	1.83	3.3489	
SUM (Σ)		7		6.8334	

Therefore, we can obtain the values of C, SE, and Z (by the formulas shown under Time-Series Analysis) as follows.

$n = 6$, SE = 0.338, C = 0.4878, and Z = 1.443 ($p = 0.0749$ is also called "Likelihood").

Keep repeating this process, we eventually are able to calculate Likelihood, Bayes Factor (the ratio of likelihoods), and posterior probability of each consecutive phases (See Questions 34 and 36 in Part I for further details.)

The following table shows a summary of the results of each phase.

Phases	Hypothesis	Prior Probability	Likelihood	Bayes Factor (λ)	Prior × Likelihood	Posterior Probability	
A_1B_1	H_o	0.5	0.0749	0.08096	0.03745	0.0749	Moderate Treatment Effect*
	H_a	0.5	0.9251		0.46255	0.9251	
B_1A_2	H_o	0.0749	0.3936	0.6491	0.0295	0.05	Weak Withdrawal Effect**
	H_a	0.9251	0.6064	0.5610	0.95		

*The strength of evidence during the first two phases showed that the first treatment is Moderate.

**The strength of evidence during the second two phases showed that the withdrawal effect is Weak.

Subject 1: Vocalizations

1. Descriptive Statistics

A_1: MEAN = 2.66, MEDIAN = 3, SD = 0.577, $n = 3$
B_1: MEAN = 5.66, MEDIAN = 5, SD = 1.154, $n = 3$
A_2: MEAN = 6.00, MEDIAN = 6, SD = 0.000, $n = 1$

Correlation Coefficients: r (A_1 and B_1) = −1.000, r (B_1 and A_2) = −0.500

μ (A_1 and B_1) = 4.17, μ(B_1 and A_2) = 5.75

2. Mann-Whitney U Test

(g) For the first two phases (A_1 and B_1)

U = 0.0, Z = 1.96, p <0.05 (Significant)

(h) For the next two phases (B_1 and A_2)

U = 1.0, Z = 0.44, p >0.05 (Not significant)

3. Time-Series Analysis

Phases	C	$Z = C/SE$	p-value	Significance
A_1	0.249	0.707	0.239	Not significant
B_1	0.249	0.707	0.239	Not significant
A_1 and B_1	0.584	1.727	0.042	Significant
A_2	0.000	0.000	0.500	Not significant

Where SE = SQR $[(n-2)/(n+1)(n-1)]$, C = $1-[\Sigma(X_i-X_i+_1)^2/2\Sigma(X-\mu)^2]$, and Z = C/SE

4. Bayesian Analysis

Hypothesis: H_o: No Effect, H_a: An Effect Exists

(i) For the first two phases (A_1 and B_1)

Data	(X_i-X_{i+1})	$(X_i-X_{i+1})^2$	$(X-\mu)$	$(X-\mu)^2$	Phases
3	0	0	−1.17	1.3689	A_1
3	1	1	−1.17	1.3689	
2	−3	9	−2.17	4.7089	
5	0	0	0.83	0.6889	B_1
5	−2	4	0.83	0.6889	
7	—	—	2.83	8.0089	
SUM (Σ)		14		16.8334	

Therefore, we can obtain the values of C, SE, and Z (by the formulas shown under Time-Series Analysis) as follows.

$n = 6$, SE = 0.338, C = 0.5842, and Z = 1.728 (p = 0.0418 is also called "Likelihood").

Keep repeating this process, we eventually are able to calculate Likelihood, Bayes Factor (the ratio of likelihoods), and posterior probability of each consecutive phases (See Questions 34 and 36 in Part I for further details.)

The following table shows a summary of the results of each phase.

Phases	Hypothesis	Prior Probability	Likelihood	Bayes Factor (λ)	Prior × Likelihood	Posterior Probability	
A_1B_1	H_o	0.5	0.0418	0.0436	0.0209	0.0418	Moderate Treatment Effect*
	H_a	0.5	0.9582		0.4791	0.9582	
B_1A_2	H_o	0.0418	0.3936	0.6491	0.01645	0.0275	Weak Withdrawal Effect **
	H_a	0.9582	0.6064		0.58105	0.9725	

*The strength of evidence during the first two phases showed that the first treatment is Moderate.

**The strength of evidence during the second two phases showed that the withdrawal effect is Weak.

Subject 2: Eye Contact

1. Descriptive Statistics

A_1: MEAN = 2.66, MEDIAN = 3, SD = 0.577, $n = 3$
B_1: MEAN = 5.00, MEDIAN = 5, SD = 0.000, $n = 3$
A_2: MEAN = 4.00, MEDIAN = 4, SD = 0.000, $n = 1$

Correlation Coefficients: r (A_1 and B_1) = 0.000, r (B_1 and A_2) = −0.000

μ (A_1 and B_1) = 3.83, μ(B_1 and A_2) = 4.75

2. Mann-Whitney U Test

(a) For the first two phases (A_1 and B_1)
    $U = 0.0$, $Z = 1.96$, $p < 0.05$ (Significant)

(b) For the next two phases (B_1 and A_2)
    $U = 0.0$, $Z = 1.34$, $p > 0.05$ (Not significant)

3. Time-Series Analysis

Phases	C	$Z = C/SE$	p-value	Significance
A_1	−0.500	−1.414	0.921	Not significant
B_1	0.000	0.000	0.500	Not significant
A_1 and B_1	0.660	1.953	0.025	Significant
A_2	0.000	0.000	0.500	Not significant

Where SE = SQR $[(n-2)/(n+1)(n-1)]$, C = $1-[\Sigma(X_i-X_i+_1)^2/2\Sigma(X-\mu)^2]$, and Z = C/SE

4. Bayesian Analysis

Hypothesis: H_o: No Effect, H_a: An Effect Exists

(c) For the first two phases (A_1 and B_1)

Data	(X_i-X_{i+1})	$(X_i-X_{i+1})^2$	$(X-\mu)$	$(X-\mu)^2$	Phases
3	1	1	−0.83	0.6889	A_1
2	−1	1	−1.83	3.3489	
3	−2	4	−0.83	0.6889	
5	0	0	1.17	1.3689	B_1
5	0	0	1.17	1.3689	
5	—	—	1.17	1.3689	
SUM (Σ)		6		8.8334	

Therefore, we can obtain the values of C, SE, and Z (by the formulas shown under Time-Series Analysis) as follows.

$n = 6$, SE = 0.338, C = 0.660, and Z = 1.953 ($p = 0.0256$ is also called "Likelihood").

Keep repeating this process, we eventually are able to calculate Likelihood, Bayes Factor (the ratio of likelihoods), and posterior probability of each consecutive phases (See Questions 34 and 36 in Part I for further details.)`

The following table shows a summary of the results of each phase.

Phases	Hypothesis	Prior Probability	Likelihood	Bayes Factor (λ)	Prior × Likelihood	Posterior Probability	
A_1B_1	H_o	0.5	0.0256	0.02627	0.0128	0.0256	Moderate to Strong Treatment Effect*
	H_a	0.5	0.9744		0.4872	0.9744	
B_1A_2	H_o	0.0256	0.1635	0.1955	0.0042	0.00513	Weak Withdrawal Effect**
	H_a	0.9744	0.8365		0.8151	0.99487	

*The strength of evidence during the first two phases showed that the first treatment is Moderate to Strong.

**The strength of evidence during the second two phases showed that the withdrawal effect is Weak.

Subject 2: Actions

1. Descriptive Statistics

A_1: MEAN = 3.33, MEDIAN = 4, SD = 1.154, $n = 3$
B_1: MEAN = 5.00, MEDIAN = 5, SD = 1, $n = 3$
A_2: MEAN = 5.00, MEDIAN = 5, SD = 0.000, $n = 1$

Correlation Coefficients: r (A_1 and B_1) = −0.866, r (B_1 and A_2) = 0.866

μ (A_1 and B_1) = 4.17, μ(B_1 and A_2) = 5

2. Mann-Whitney U Test

(d) For the first two phases (A_1 and B_1)

   U = 1.0, Z = 1.52, p >0.05 (Not significant)

(e) For the next two phases (B_1 and A_2)

   U = 1.5, Z = 0.00, p >0.05 (Not significant)

3. Time-Series Analysis

Phases	C	$Z = C/SE$	p-value	Significance
A_1	0.249	0.707	0.239	Not significant
B_1	−0.250	−0.707	0.760	Not significant
A_1 and B_1	0.264	0.781	0.217	Not significant
A_2	0.000	0.000	0.500	Not significant

Where SE = SQR $[(n-2)/(n+1)(n-1)]$, C = $1-[\Sigma(X_i-X_i+_1)^2/2\Sigma(X-\mu)^2]$, and Z = C/SE

4. Bayesian Analysis

Hypothesis: H_o: No Effect, H_a: An Effect Exists

(f) For the first two phases (A_1 and B_1)

Data	(X_i-X_{i+1})	$(X_i-X_{i+1})^2$	$(X-\mu)$	$(X-\mu)^2$	Phases
2	−2	4	−2.17	4.7089	A_1
4	0	0	−0.17	0.0289	
4	−2	4	−0.17	0.0289	
6	2	4	1.83	3.3489	B_1
4	−1	1	−0.17	0.0289	
5	—	—	0.83	0.6889	
SUM (Σ)		13		8.8334	

Therefore, we can obtain the values of C, SE, and Z (by the formulas shown under Time-Series Analysis) as follows.

$n = 6$, SE $= 0.338$, C $= 0.264$, and Z $= 0.78$ ($p = 0.2177$ is also called "Likelihood").

Keep repeating this process, we eventually are able to calculate Likelihood, Bayes Factor (the ratio of likelihoods), and posterior probability of each consecutive phases (See Questions 34 and 36 in Part I for further details.)

The following table shows a summary of the results of each phase.

Phases	Hypothesis	Prior Probability	Likelihood	Bayes Factor (λ)	Prior × Likelihood	Posterior Probability	
A_1B_1	H_o	0.5	0.2177	0.278	0.10885	0.2177	Weak Treatment Effect*
	H_a	0.5	0.7823		0.39115	0.7823	
B_1A_2	H_o	0.2177	0.7704	3.355	0.01677	0.0854	Weak Withdrawal Effect**
	H_a	0.7823	0.2296		0.17962	0.9146	

*The strength of evidence during the first two phases showed that the first treatment is Weak.

**The strength of evidence during the second two phases showed that the withdrawal effect is Weak.

Subject 2: Vocalizations

1. Descriptive Statistics

A_1: MEAN = 3.33, MEDIAN = 3, SD = 1.527, $n = 3$
B_1: MEAN = 5.00, MEDIAN = 5, SD = 1.000, $n = 3$
A_2: MEAN = 5.00, MEDIAN = 5, SD = 0, $n = 1$

Correlation Coefficients: r (A_1 and B_1) = −0.327, r (B_1 and A_2) = −0.866

μ (A_1 and B_1)= 4.17, μ(B_1 and A_2)= 5

2. Mann-Whitney U Test

(g) For the first two phases (A_1 and B_1)

U = 1.5, Z = 1.30, p >0.05 (Not significant)

(h) For the next two phases (B_1 and A_2)

U = 1.5, Z = 0.00, p >0.05 (Not significant)

3. Time-Series Analysis

Phases	C	$Z = C/SE$	p-value	Significance
A_1	−0.392	−1.111	0.866	Not significant
B_1	0.500	1.414	0.078	Not significant
A_1 and B_1	0.123	0.364	0.357	Not significant
A_2	0.000	0.000	0.500	Not significant

Where $SE = SQR\ [(n-2)/(n+1)(n-1)]$, $C = 1-[\Sigma(X_i-X_i+_1)^2/2\Sigma(X-\mu)^2]$, and $Z = C/SE$

4. Bayesian Analysis

Hypothesis: H_o: No Effect, H_a: An Effect Exists

(i) For the first two phases (A_1 and B_1)

Data	(X_i-X_{i+1})	$(X_i-X_{i+1})^2$	$(X-\mu)$	$(X-\mu)^2$	Phases
3	−2	4	−1.17	1.3689	A_1
5	3	9	0.83	0.6889	
2	−2	4	−2.17	4.7089	
4	−1	1	−0.17	0.0289	B_1
5	−1	1	0.83	0.6889	
6	—	—	1.83	3.3489	
SUM (Σ)		19		10.8334	

Therefore, we can obtain the values of C, SE, and Z (by the formulas shown under Time-Series Analysis) as follows.

N = 6, SE = 0.338, C = 0.123, and Z = 0.364 ($p = 0.3594$ is also called "Likelihood").

Keep repeating this process, we eventually are able to calculate Likelihood, Bayes Factor (the ratio of likelihoods), and posterior probability of each consecutive phases (See Questions 34 and 36 in Part I for further details.)

The following table shows a summary of the results of each phase.

Phases	Hypothesis	Prior Probability	Likelihood	Bayes Factor (λ)	Prior × Likelihood	Posterior Probability	
A_1B_1	H_o	0.5	0.3594	0.5610	0.1797	0.3594	Weak Treatment Effect*
	H_a	0.5	0.6406		0.3203	0.6406	
B_1A_2	H_o	0.3594	0.2296	0.298	0.08252	0.14325	Weak Withdrawal Effect**
	H_a	0.6406	0.7704		0.49352	0.85675	

*The strength of evidence during the first two phases showed that the first treatment is Weak.
**The strength of evidence during the second two phases showed that the withdrawal effect is Weak.

Subject 3: Eye Contact

1. Descriptive Statistics

A_1: MEAN = 1.66, MEDIAN = 2, SD = 0.577, $n = 3$
B_1: MEAN = 2.66, MEDIAN = 2, SD = 1.154, $n = 3$
A_2: MEAN = 3.00, MEDIAN = 3, SD = 0.000, $n = 1$

Correlation Coefficients: r (A_1 and B_1) = 0.500, r (B_1 and A_2) = –0.500

μ (A_1 and B_1) = 2.17, μ(B_1 and A_2) = 2.75

2. Mann-Whitney U Test

(a) For the first two phases (A_1 and B_1)
   U = 2.0, = 1.09, p >0.05 (Not significant)

(b) For the next two phases (B_1 and A_2)
   U = 1.0, Z = 0.44, p >0.05 (Not significant)

3. Time-Series Analysis

Phases	C	$Z = C/SE$	p-value	Significance
A_1	–0.500	–1.414	0.921	Not significant
B_1	0.249	0.707	0.239	Not significant
A_1 and B_1	0.379	1.122	0.131	Not significant
A_2	0.000	0.000	0.500	Not significant

Where SE = SQR $[(n-2)/(n+1)(n-1)]$, C = $1-[\Sigma(X_i-X_i+_1)^2/2\Sigma(X-\mu)^2]$, and Z = C/SE

4. Bayesian Analysis

Hypothesis: H_0: No Effect, H_a: An Effect Exists

(c) For the first two phases (A_1 and B_1)

Data	$(X_i - X_{i+1})$	$(X_i - X_{i+1})^2$	$(X - \mu)$	$(X - \mu)^2$	Phases
2	1	1	−0.17	0.0289	A_1
1	−1	1	−1.17	1.3689	
2	0	0	−0.17	0.0289	
2	0	0	−0.17	0.0289	B_1
2	−2	4	−0.17	0.0289	
4	—	—	1.83	3.3489	
SUM (Σ)		6		4.8334	

Therefore, we can obtain the values of C, SE, and Z (by the formulas shown under Time-Series Analysis) as follows.

$n = 6$, SE = 0.338, C = 0.3793, and Z = 1.122 ($p = 0.1314$ is also called "Likelihood").

Keep repeating this process, we eventually are able to calculate Likelihood, Bayes Factor (the ratio of likelihoods), and posterior probability of each consecutive phases (See Questions 34 and 36 in Part I for further details.)

The following table shows a summary of the results of each phase.

Phases	Hypothesis	Prior Probability	Likelihood	Bayes Factor (λ)	Prior × Likelihood	Posterior Probability	
A_1B_1	H_0	0.5	0.1314	0.1512	0.0657	0.1314	Weak to Moderate Treatment Effect*
	H_a	0.5	0.8686		0.4343	0.8686	
B_1A_2	H_0	0.1314	0.3936	0.649	0.05172	0.08941	Weak Withdrawal Effect**
	H_a	0.8686	0.6064		0.52672	0.91059	

*The strength of evidence during the first two phases showed that the first treatment is Weak to Moderate.

**The strength of evidence during the second two phases showed that the withdrawal effect is Weak.

Subject 3: Actions

1. Descriptive Statistics

A_1: MEAN = 2.33, MEDIAN = 2, SD = 0.577, $n = 3$
B_1: MEAN = 3.00, MEDIAN = 3, SD = 1.000, $n = 3$
A_2: MEAN = 4.00, MEDIAN = 4, SD = 0.000, $n = 1$

Correlation Coefficients: r (A_1 and B_1) = 0.000, r (B_1 and A_2) = 0.866

μ (A_1 and B_1) = 2.67, μ(B_1 and A_2) = 3.25

2. Mann-Whitney U Test

(d) For the first two phases (A_1 and B_1)
    U = 2.5, Z = 0.87, p >0.05 (Not significant)

(e) For the next two phases (B_1 and A_2)
    U = 0.5, Z = 0.89, p >0.05 (Not significant)

3. Time-Series Analysis

Phases	C	$Z = C/SE$	p-value	Significance
A_1	0.249	0.707	0.239	Not significant
B_1	−0.250	−0.707	0.760	Not significant
A_1 and B_1	−0.049	−0.147	0.558	Not significant
A_2	0.000	0.000	0.500	Not significant

Where SE = SQR $[(n-2)/(n+1)(n-1)]$, C = $1-[\Sigma(X_i-X_i+_1)^2/2\Sigma(X-\mu)^2]$, and Z = C/SE

4. Bayesian Analysis

Hypothesis: H_0: No Effect, H_a: An Effect Exists

(f) For the first two phases (A_1 and B_1)

Data	(X_i-X_{i+1})	$(X_i-X_{i+1})^2$	$(X-\mu)$	$(X-\mu)^2$	Phases
2	0	0	−0.67	0.4489	A_1
2	−1	1	−0.67	0.4489	
3	−1	1	0.33	0.1089	
4	2	4	1.33	1.7689	B_1
2	−1	1	−0.67	0.4489	
3	—	—	0.33	0.1089	
SUM (Σ)		7		3.3334	

Therefore, we can obtain the values of C, SE, and Z (by the formulas shown under Time-Series Analysis) as follows.

$n = 6$, SE = 0.338, C = −0.05, and Z = −0.148 (p = 0.5596 is also called "Likelihood").

Keep repeating this process, we will eventually be able to calculate Likelihood, Bayes Factor (the ratio of likelihoods), and posterior probability of each consecutive phases (See Questions 34 and 36 in Part I for further details.)

The following table shows a summary of the results of each phase.

Phases	Hypothesis	Prior Probability	Likelihood	Bayes Factor (λ)	Prior × Likelihood	Posterior Probability	
A_1B_1	H_o	0.5	0.5596	1.27	0.2798	0.5596	Weak Treatment Effect*
	H_a	0.5	0.4404		0.2202	0.4404	
B_1A_2	H_o	0.5596	0.6064	1.54	0.33934	0.66189	Weak Withdrawal Effect**
	H_a	0.4404	0.3936		0.17334	0.33811	

*The strength of evidence during the first two phases showed that the first treatment is Weak.

**The strength of evidence during the second two phases showed that the withdrawal effect is Weak.

Subject 3: Vocalizations

1. Descriptive Statistics

A_1: MEAN = 1.33, MEDIAN = 1, SD = 0.577, $n = 3$
B_1: MEAN = 2.33, MEDIAN = 2, SD = 0.577, $n = 3$
A_2: MEAN = 3.00, MEDIAN = 3, SD = 0.000, $n = 1$

Correlation Coefficients: r (A_1 and B_1) = 1.000, r (B_1 and A_2) = −0.500

μ (A_1 and B_1) = 1.83, μ(B_1 and A_2) = 2.500

2. Mann-Whitney U Test

(g) For the first two phases (A_1 and B_1)

U = 1.0, Z = 1.52, p >0.05 (Not significant)

(h) For the next two phases (B_1 and A_2)

U = 0.5, Z = 0.89, p >0.05 (Not significant)

3. Time-Series Analysis

Phases	C	$Z = C/SE$	p-value	Significance
A_1	−0.500	−1.414	0.921	Not significant
B_1	−0.500	−1.414	0.921	Not significant
A_1 and B_1	0.117	0.348	0.363	Not significant
A_2	0.000	0.000	0.500	Not significant

Where SE = SQR $[(n-2)/(n+1)(n-1)]$, C = $1-[\Sigma(X_i-X_i+_1)^2/2\Sigma(X-\mu)^2]$, and Z = C/SE

4. Bayesian Analysis

Hypothesis: H_o: No Effect, H_a: An Effect Exists

(i)   For the first two phases (A_1 and B_1)

Data	(X_i-X_{i+1})	$(X_i-X_{i+1})^2$	$(X-\mu)$	$(X-\mu)^2$	Phases
1	−1	1	−0.83	0.6889	A_1
2	1	1	0.17	0.0289	
1	−1	1	−0.83	0.6889	
2	−1	1	0.17	0.0289	B_1
3	1	1	1.17	1.3689	
2	—	—	0.17	0.0289	
SUM (Σ)		5		10.8334	

Therefore, we can obtain the values of C, SE, and Z (by the formulas shown under Time-Series Analysis) as follows.

$n = 6$, SE = 0.338, C = 0.118, and Z = 0.348 ($p = 0.3632$ is also called "Likelihood").

Keep repeating this process, we eventually are able to calculate Likelihood, Bayes Factor (the ratio of likelihoods), and posterior probability of each consecutive phases (See Questions 34 and 36 in Part I for further details.)

The following table shows a summary of the results of each phase.

Phases	Hypothesis	Prior Probability	Likelihood	Bayes Factor (λ)	Prior × Likelihood	Posterior Probability	
A_1B_1	H_o	0.5	0.3632	0.57	0.1816	0.3632	Weak Treatment Effect*
	H_a	0.5	0.6368		0.3184	0.6368	
B_1A_2	H_o	0.3632	0.9306	13.41	0.3380	0.88435	Very Weak Withdrawal Effect**
	H_a	0.6368	0.0694		0.0442	0.11565	

*The strength of evidence during the first two phases showed that the first treatment is Weak.

**The strength of evidence during the second two phases showed that the withdrawal effect is Very Weak.

APPENDIX

Analysis of Single Subject Data Using the Beta Probability Distribution

(for mathematically inclined readers)

Bayesian Approach with Beta Distribution: A Hypothetical Example in A-B Design

---

Given the following set of hypothetical data values in A-B design, we will derive the maximum likelihood (a.k.a. Bayesian *p*-value) of a subject's score change day-to-day to determine the strength of evidence.

A_1: 5, 4, 4, 2, 3, 4, 4, 6 (out of 10)

B_1: 7, 5, 4, 6, 6, 7, 5, 4, 7, 7 (out of 10)

It is mathematically convenient for us to convert each score into its decimal equivalent, so that we now have:

A_1: 0.5, 0.4, 0.4, 0.2, 0.3, 0.4, 0.4, 0.6

B_1: 0.7, 0.5, 0.4, 0.6, 0.6, 0.7, 0.5, 0.4, 0.7, 0.7

Using the formulas in Question 35 of Part I, we calculate as follows:

A_1: $\mu (A_1) = 0.4$, $\sigma^2(A_1) = 0.125$, a =
$\mu [(\mu \times (1-\mu)/s^2) -1] = 0.368$,
$B = (1-\mu)[(\mu \times (1-\mu)/\sigma^2) -1] = 0.552$,
$\mu = (a+x)/(a+b+n)$,
$\sigma^2 = [\mu \times (1-\mu)/(a+b+n+1)$

B_1: 1st value = 0.7, so that the cumulative density function F (X) can be calculated P(X = 0.7, given that B (0.368, 0.552) is provided) as follows:
$F (0<X<0.7) = \int^{0.7} [t^{0.368-1} \times (1-t)^{0.552-1}]/ B (0.368, 0.552) = 0.72774$

The Bayesian *p*-value is given as $1-F (X) = 1-0.72774 = 0.27226$; therefore, after the 1st day of Intervention period, we did not detect a significant treatment effect ($p>0.05$). The software packages such as MINITAB 14 or SPSS can easily derive the calculation shown above.

By the same token, we have a 2nd value 0.5, so that we calculate a and b for the new Beta density function B (a, b) such that

$\mu = (0.368 + 0.7)/(0.368 + 0.552 + 1) = 0.55625,$

$\sigma = \text{SQR } [(0.55625) \times (1-0.55625)/(0.368+0.552+1+1)] = 0.17$, where $n = 1$ and $x = 0.7$,

$a = 1.06805$, $b = 0.85204$, and F $(0<X<0.5) = $ F $(0.5) = 0.42330$

Therefore, the Bayesian p-value after Day 2 is 0.57670 (1–0.42330). Again, we did not detect a significant treatment effect. The p-value after Day 2 is actually larger than the one after Day 1, so the strength of evidence of the treatment got weaker by almost 30%.

Keep repeating this process to update the maximum likelihood of a treatment efficacy in each of the 11 days, and then we can obtain the following results (Table AP-1).

Figures AP-1 through AP-10 show the beta distribution curve of each trial graphically. As can be seen in the figures, the interval for probability density distribution gets narrower and, for larger values of a and b, the distributions are seen to have less spread or variance and are relatively more peaked. Prior specification of beta distribution with larger a and b corresponds to having more information (messages), or a more precise view initially, about the true population parameter of interest than in the case that a and b are smaller. It means that the maximum likelihood of μ (the central value of the probability density distribution) converges to a true population mean μ. Technically, the beta distribution shown is a continuous distribution, for which the total area under the beta curve is 100%. The height of the beta curve is described as the probability density for the parameter values and the distribution function represents the cumulative probabilities of the random variable.

The Bayesian capacity to accommodate continuous revision of a probability from one behavioral act to the next makes it quite suitable for detecting and determining a subject's behavioral change from a variety of perspectives in which prediction is an important factor. The cumulative treatment of the data from behavioral shift to behavioral shift adjusts the margin of error and increases the predictability of the final results (Amato & Satake, 2007). Theoretically, through beta distribution, the predictability of the parameter of interest will increase as new empirical data emerge (Maxwell & Satake, 1997, 2005).

Both the Bayesian and classical methods to statistical inference are typical ways of conducting hypothesis testing. Each method should be viewed as a mere tool in a tool kit. More specifically, a clinical practitioner should retain the freedom to choose and apply whichever method is most suitable in answering the research questions.

Predicting the future is always risky business and a Bayesian analysis does not reduce or remove the risk. As with classical statistics, the analyses and interpretations of beta probabilities are complicated by the factors that go into any measure of human behavior. Nevertheless, prediction is dependent on the statistical nature of human behavior and, as noted earlier, Bayesian statistical methodologies are more suitable with process-oriented phenomena than classical statistical methodologies (Satake, 1994).

Table AP–1. Summary of Beta (a, b) in Each of 11 Days

Intervention (B₁)	Data Values	μ	σ	Beta (a,b)	F(X)	P-value 1–F(X)	Change (+ or –)
Day 1	0.7	0.5563	0.17	(0.37, 0.55)	0.7277	0.2723	
Day 2	0.5	0.5370	0.2518	(1.07, 0.85)	0.4233	0.5767	–0.304
Day 3	0.4	0.5021	0.2254	(1.57, 1.35)	0.3214	0.6786	–0.1020
Day 4	0.6	0.5220	0.2053	(1.97, 1.95)	0.6430	0.3570	+0.322
Day 5	0.6	0.5352	0.1896	(2.57, 2.35)	0.6253	0.3747	–0.0177
Day 6	0.7	0.5590	0.1764	(3.17, 2.75)	0.7846	0.2154	+0.159
Day 7	0.5	0.5515	0.1665	(3.87, 3.05)	0.3706	0.6294	–0.414
Day 8	0.4	0.5345	0.1584	(4.37, 3.55)	0.1956	0.8044	–0.175
Day 9	0.7	0.5512	0.1505	(4.77, 4.15)	0.8398	0.1602	+0.644
Day 10	0.7	—	—	(5.47, 4.45)	0.8264	0.1736	–0.0134
Day 11	x	—	—				

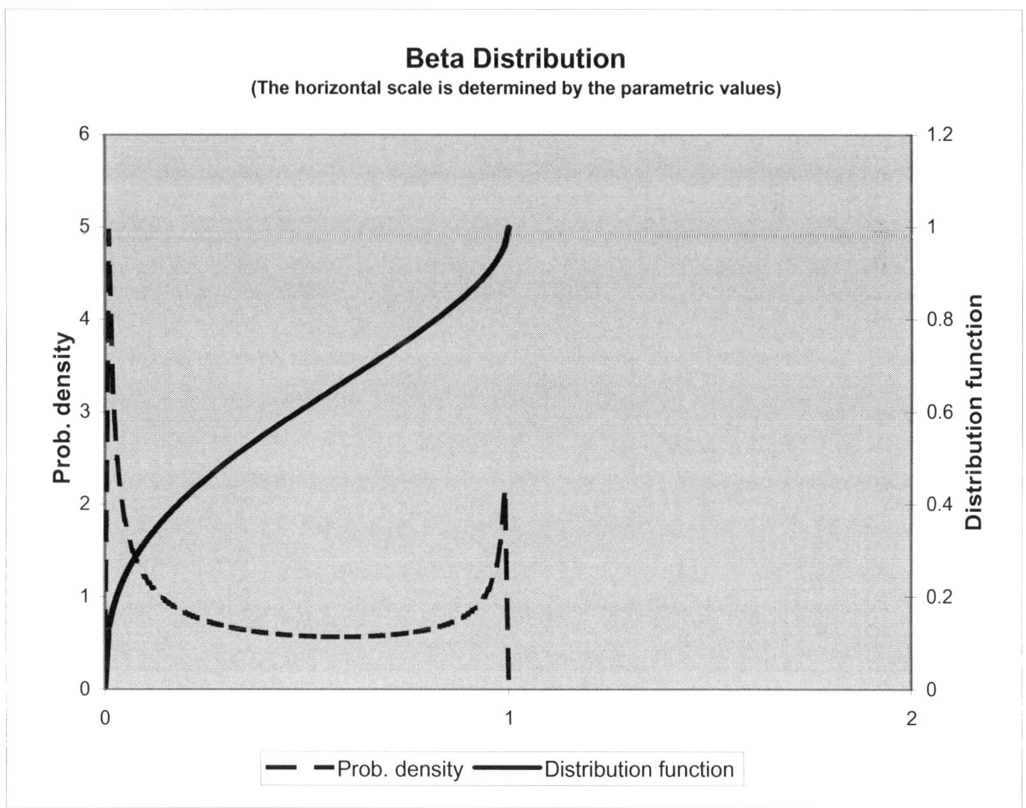

Figure AP–1. Beta Graph of Day 1.

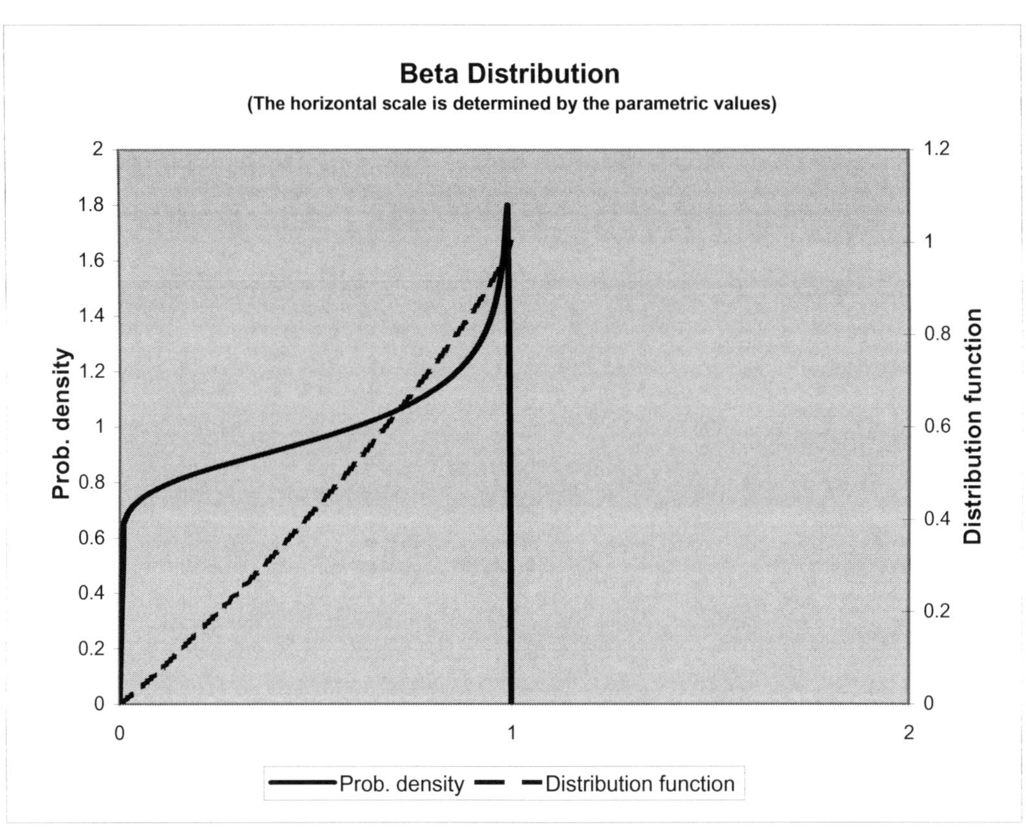

Figure AP–2. Beta Graph of Day 2.

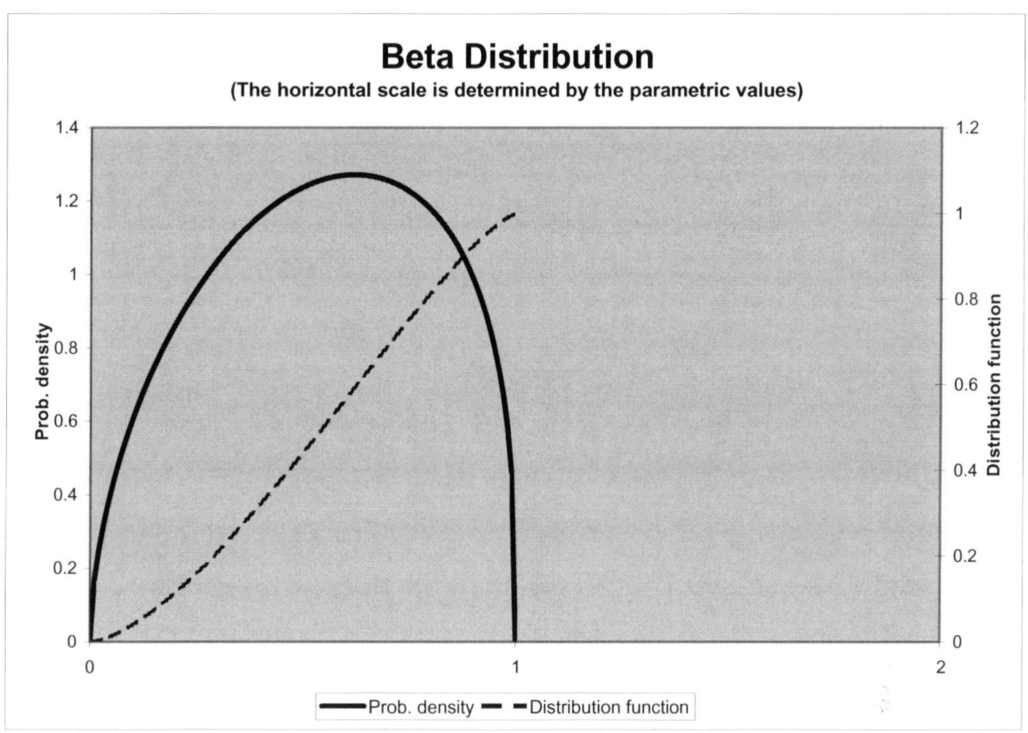

Figure AP–3. Beta Graph of Day 3.

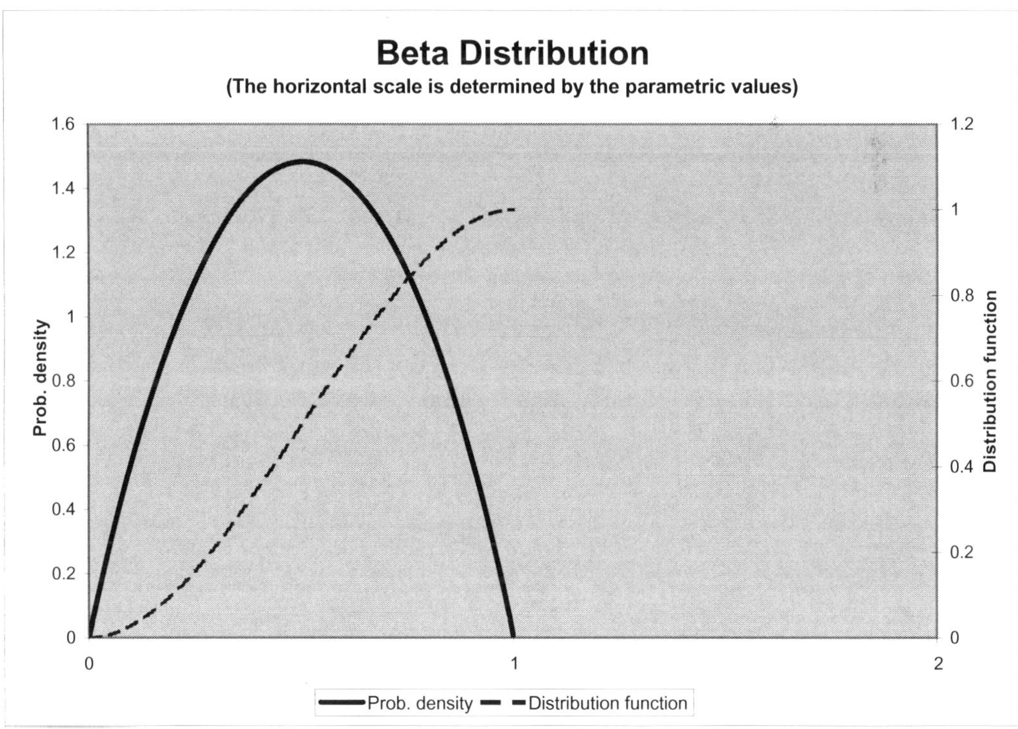

Figure AP–4. Beta Graph of Day 4.

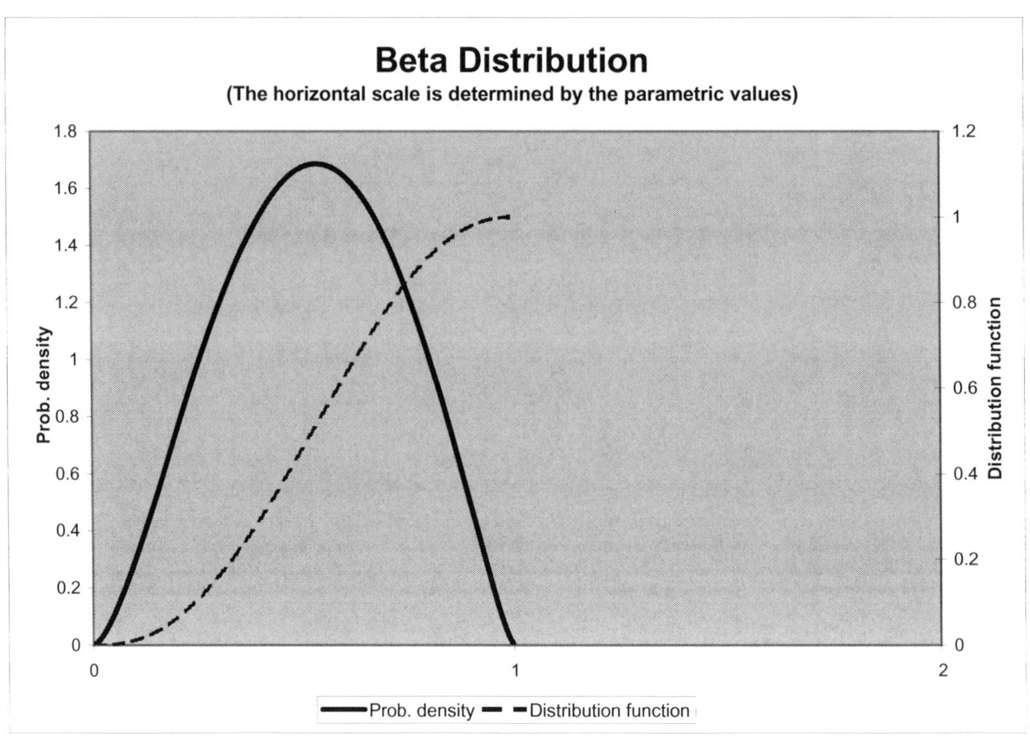

Figure AP–5. Beta Graph of Day 5.

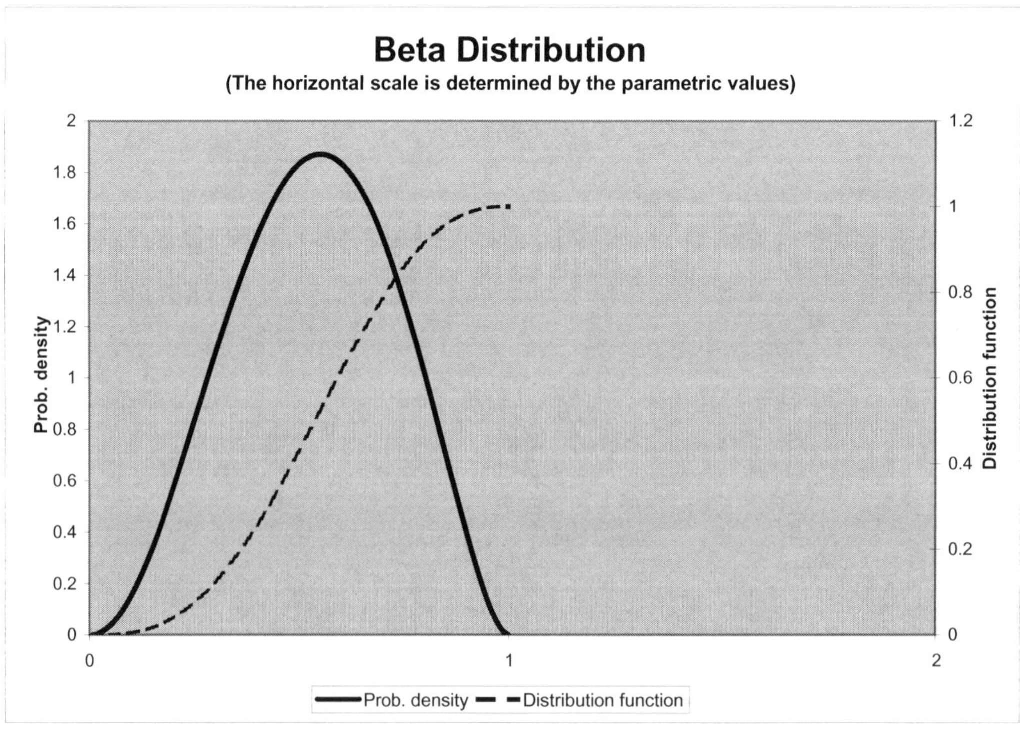

Figure AP–6. Beta Graph of Day 6.

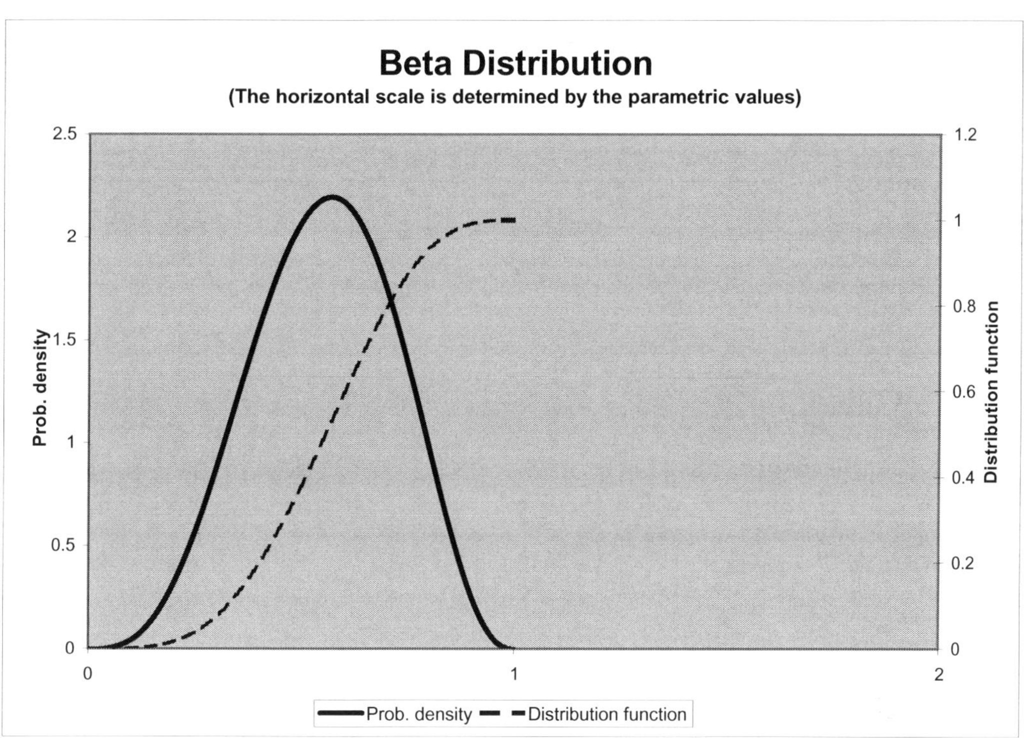

Figure AP–7. Beta Graph of Day 7.

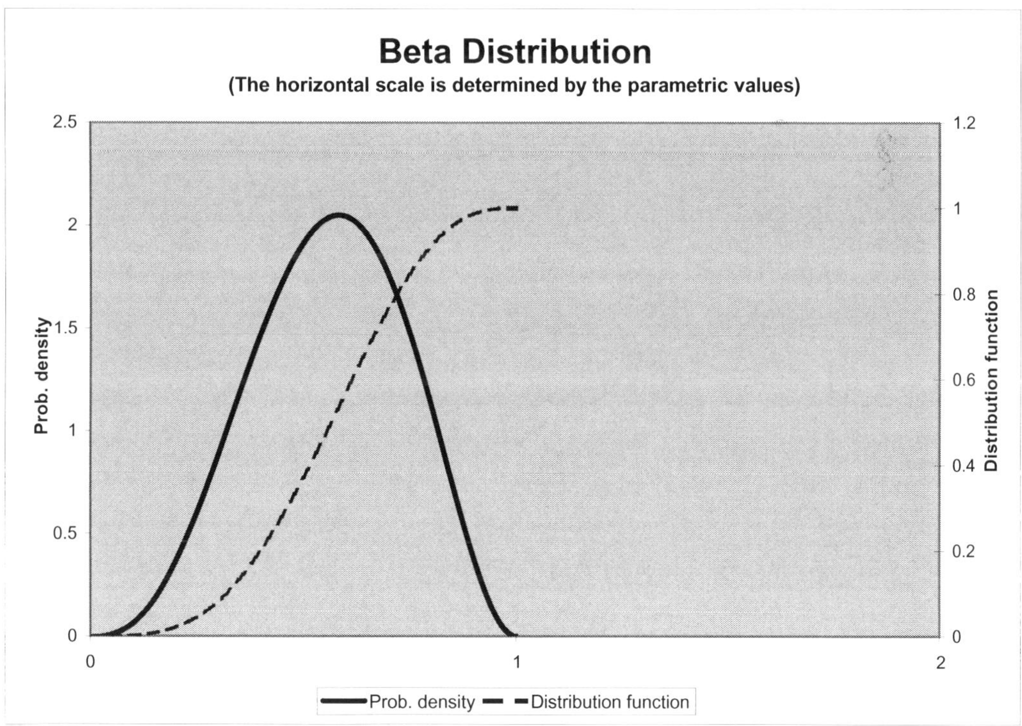

Figure AP–8. Beta Graph of Day 8.

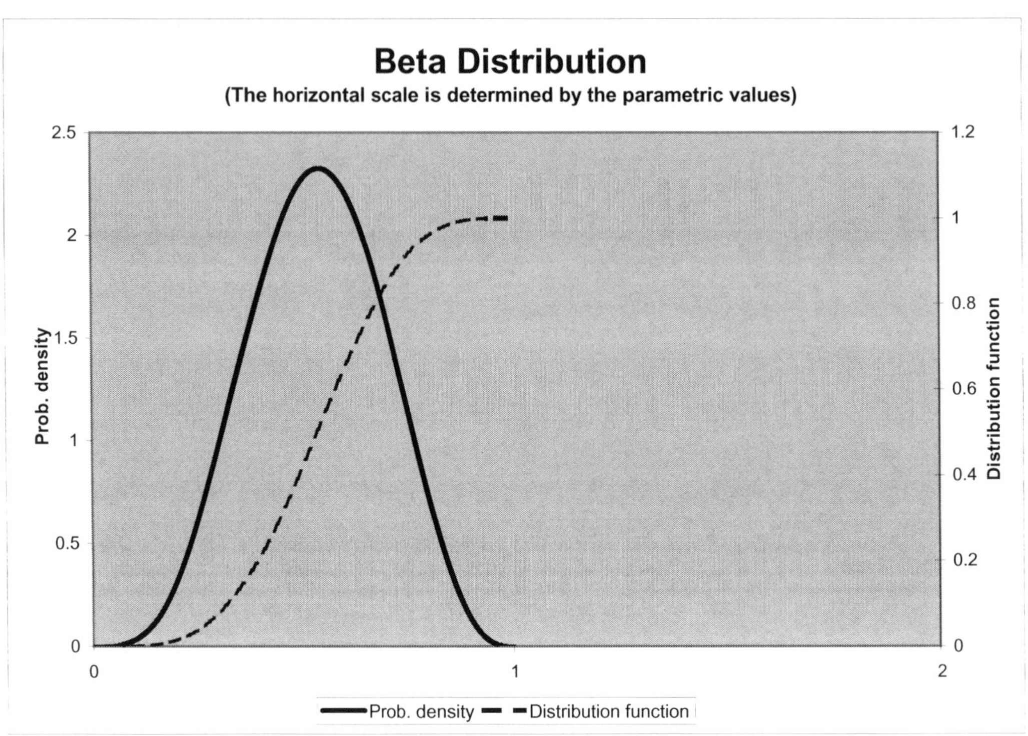

Figure AP–9. Beta Graph of Day 9.

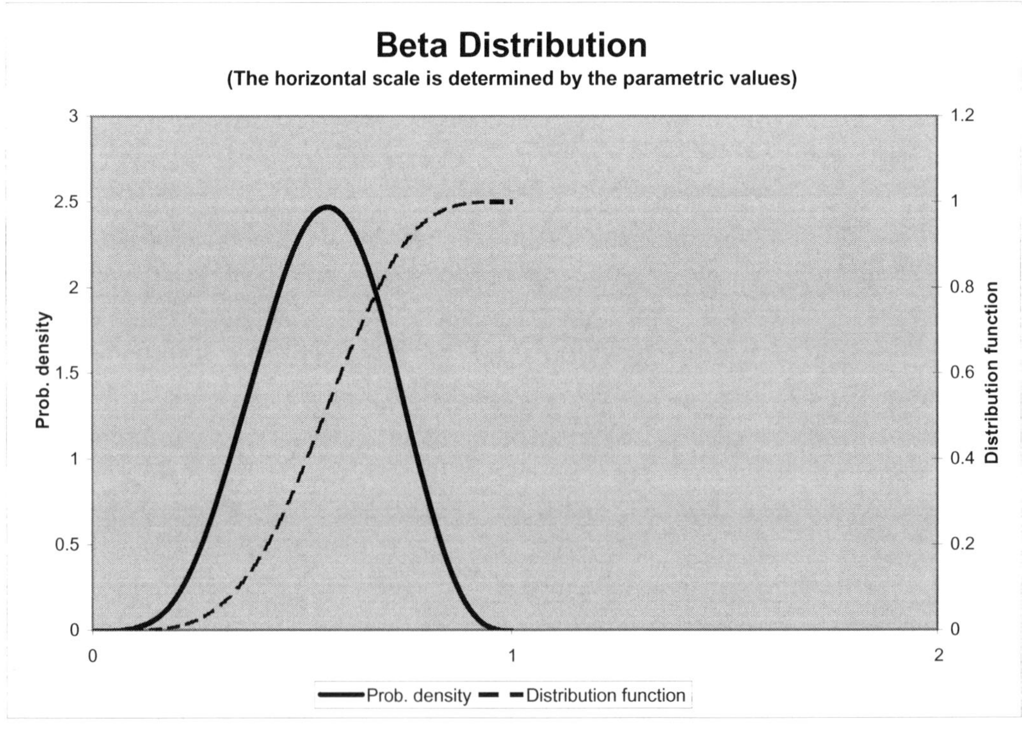

Figure AP–10. Beta Graph of Day 10.

References

Amato, P. P., & Satake, E. (2007). A Bayesian model of interpersonal transactions in a business setting. *International Academy of Business Discipline Research Year Book*, Vol 1.

Barlow, D. H., Hayes, S. C., & Nelson, R. O. (1984). *The scientist practitioner: Research and accountability in clinical and educational settings.* Oxford: Pergamon Press.

Barlow, D. H., & Hersen, M. (1984). *Single case experimental designs.* New York: Pergamon Press.

Baron-Cohen, S., Tager-Flusberg, H., & Cohen, D. J. (2000). *Understanding other minds: Perspectives from developmental cognitive neuroscience* (2nd ed.). Oxford: Oxford University Press.

Bernabei, P., & Camaioni, L. (2001). Developmental profile and regression in a child with autism: A single case study. *Autism, 5*(3), 1362–3613.

Callahan, C. D., & Barisa, M. T. (2005). Statistical process control and rehabilitation outcome: The single-subject design reconsidered. *Rehabilitation Psychology, 50*(1), 24–33.

Caplan, D. (2003) Aphasic syndromes. In K. M. Heilman & E. Valenstein (Eds.), *Clinical neuropsychology* (4th ed., pp. 14–34). New York: Oxford University Press.

Case-Smith, J., & Bryan, T. (1999). The effects of occupational therapy with sensory integration emphasis on preschool-age children with autism. *American Journal of Occupational Therapy, 53*(5), 489–497.

Charman, T. Baron-Cohen, S., Swettenham, J., Baird, G., Drew, A., & Cox, A. (2003). Predicting language outcomes in infants with autism and pervasive developmental disorder. *International Journal of Language and Communication Disorders, 38*(3), 265–285.

Charman, T., Swettenham, J., Baron-Cohen, S., Cox, A., Baird, G., & Drew, A. (1997). Infants with autism: An investigation of empathy, pretend play, joint attention, and imitation. *Developmental Psychology, 33*(5), 781–789.

Clare, L., Wilson, B. A., Carter, G., & Hodges, J. R. (2003). Cognitive rehabilitation as a component of early intervention in Alzheimer's disease: A single case study. *Aging and Mental Health, 7*(1), 15–21.

Cook, T. D., & Campbell, D. T. (1979). *Quasi-experimentation.* Chicago: Rand McNally.

Cooper, H. R., & Craddock, L. C. (2006). *Cochlear implants: A practical guide* (2nd ed.). West Sussex: Whurr.

Crosbie, J. (1993). Interrupted time-series analysis with brief single-subject data. *Journal of Consulting and Clinical Psychology, 61*, 966–974.

Cullington, H. E. (2003). *Cochlear implants: Objective measures.* Philadelphia: Whurr.

Drew, A., Baird, G., Baron-Cohen, S., Cox, A., Slonims, V., Wheelwright, S., et al. (2002). A pilot randomized control trial of a parent training intervention for pre-school children with autism: Preliminary findings and methodological challenges. *European Child and Adolescent Psychiatry, 11*, 266–272.

Duffy, J. R. (1995). *Motor speech disorders: Substrates, differential diagnosis, and management.* St. Louis, MO: Mosby.

Edgington, E. S., (1987). Randomized single-subject experiments and statistical tests. *Journal of Counseling Psychology, 34*(4), 437–442.

Fonagy, P., & Moran, G. S. (1990). Studies on the efficacy of child psychoanalysis. *Journal of Consulting and Clinical Psychology, 58*(6), 684–695.

Freed, D., Celery, K., & Marshall, R. C. (2004). Effectiveness of personalized and phonological cueing on long-term naming performance by aphasic subjects: A clinical investigation. *Aphasiology, 18*(8), 743–757.

Fridriksson, J., Holland, A. L., Beeson, P., & Morrow, L. (2005). Spaced retrieval treatment of anomia. *Aphasiology, 19*(2), 99–109.

Frith, U., & Hill, E. L. (2004). *Autism: Mind and Brain.* New York: Oxford University Press.

Fryauf-Bertschy, H., Tyler, R. S., Kelsay, D. M., Gantz, B. J., & Woodworth, G. G. (1997). Cochlear implant use by prelingually deafened children: The influences of age at implant and length of device use. *Journal of Speech, Language, and Hearing Research, 40*(1), 183–199.

Fucetola, R., Tucker, F., Blank, K., & Corbetta, M. (2005). A process for translating evidence-based aphasia treatment into clinical practice. *Aphasiology, 19*(3), 411–422.

Galassi, J. P., & Gersh, T. L. (1993). Myths, misconceptions, and missed opportunity: Single-case designs and counseling psychology. *Journal of Counseling Psychology, 40*(4), 525–531.

Gantz, B. J., & Turner, C. (2004). Combining acoustic and electrical speech processing: Iowa/Nucleus Hybrid implant. *Acta Otolaryngolica., 124*, 344–347.

Goodman, S. N. (1999). Toward evidence-based medical statistics 2: The Bayes factor. *Annals of Internal Medicine, 130*(2), 1005–1013.

Havstam, C., Buchholz, M., & Hartelius, L. (2003). Speech recognition and dysarthria: A single subject study of two individuals with profound impairment of speech and motor control. *Logopedics Phoniatrics Vocology, 28*, 81–90.

Higgins, M. B., McCleary, E. A., & Schulte, L. (1999). Altered phonatory physiology with short-term deactivation of children's cochlear implants. *Ear and Hearing, 20*(5), 426–438.

Iversen, G. R. (1984). *Bayesian statistical inference.* Newbury Park, CA: Sage.

Iyer, S. N., Rothmann, T. L., Vogler, J. E., & Spaulding, W. D. (2005). Evaluating outcomes of rehabilitation for severe mental illness. *Rehabilitation Psychology, 50*(1), 43–55.

Jones, P. W. (2003). Single-case time series with Bayesian analysis: A practitioner's guide. *Measurement and Evaluation in Counseling and Development, 36*, 28–39.

Kaye, M. S. (2000). *Guide to dysarthria management: A client-clinician approach.* Eau Claire, WI: Thinking Publications.

Kazdin, A. E. (1982). *Single-case research designs: Methods for clinical and applied setting.* New York: Oxford University Press.

Kearns, K. P. (2000). Single-subject experimental designs and treatment research. In L. J. Gonzalez-Rothi, B. Crosson, & S. E. Nadeau (Eds.), *Aphasia and language: Theory to practice* (pp. 421–441). New York: Guilford.

Kiran, S., & Thompson, C. K. (2003). The role of semantic complexity in treatment of naming deficits: Training semantic categories in fluent aphasia by controlling exemplar typicality. *Journal of Speech, Language, and Hearing Research, 46*, 773–787.

Kupper, Z. & Tschacher, W. (2002). Symptom trajectories in psychotic episodes. *Comprehensive Psychiatry, 43*(4), 311–318.

Leder, S. B., Spitzer, J. B., & Kirchner, J. C. (1987). Immediate effects of cochlear implantation on voice quality. *Archives of Oto-Rhino-Laryngology, 244*(2), 93–95.

Linebaugh, C. W., Shisler, R. J., & Lehner, L. (2005). Cueing hierarchies and word retrieval: A therapy program. *Aphasiology, 19*(1), 77–92.

Maher, C. A. (1985). Training school psychological services directors in organizational behavior management. *Professional Psychology: Research and Practice, 16*(2), 209–225.

Maxwell, D. L., & Satake, E. (1997). *Research and statistical methods in communication disorders.* Baltimore: Williams & Wilkins.

Maxwell, D. L., & Satake, E. (2006). *Research and statistical methods in communication sciences and disorders*. Clifton Park, NY: Delmar Thomson Learning.

McReynolds, L. V., & Thompson, C. K. (1986). Flexibility of single-subject experimental designs: Pt. I. Review of the basics of single-subject design. *Journal of Speech and Hearing Disorders, 51*, 194–203.

Miyamoto, R. T., Kirk, K. I., Renshaw, J., & Hussain, D. (1999). Cochlear implantation in auditory neuropathy. *Laryngoscope, 109*, 181–185.

Miyamoto, R. T., Osberger, M. J., Robbins, A. M., Myres, W. A., Kessler, K., & Pope, M. L. (1991). Comparison of speech perception abilities in deaf children with hearing aids or cochlear implants. *Otolaryngology-Head And Neck Surgery, 104*(1), 42–46.

Morrow, K. L., & Fridriksson, J. (2006). Comparing fixed- and randomized-interval spaced retrieval in anomia treatment. *Journal of Communication Disorders, 39*, 2–11.

Mundy, P., Sigman, M., Ungerer, J., & Sherman, T. (1986). Defining the social deficits of autism: The contribution of non-verbal communication measures. *Journal of Child Psychology and Psychiatry, 27*, 657–669.

Murdoch, B. E., Pitt, G., Theodoros, D. G., & Ward, E. C. (1999). Real-time continuous visual biofeedback in the treatment of speech breathing disorders following childhood traumatic brain injury: Report of one case. *Pediatric Rehabilitation, 3*(1), 5–20.

Murphy, K. P. (2000). In praise of Bayes. Retreived August 10, 2002, from http://www.cs.berkeley.edu/~murphyk/Bayes/economist.html .

Osberger, M. J., Miyamoto, R. T., Zimmerman-Phillips, S., Kemink, J. L., Stroer, B. S., Firszt, J. B., et al. (1991). Independent evaluation of the speech perception abilities of children with the Nucleus 22-channel cochlear implant system. *Ear and Hearing, 12*(Suppl. 4), 66S–80S.

Osberger, M. J., Todd, S. L., Berry, S. W., Robbins, A. M., & Miyamoto, R. T. (1991). Effect of age at onset of deafness on children's speech perception abilities with a cochlear implant. *Annals of Otology, Rhinology, and Laryngology, 100*(11), 883–888.

Ottenbacher, K. (1986). *Evaluating clinical change: Strategies for occupational and physical therapists*. Baltimore: Williams & Wilkins.

Ottenbacher, K. J., (1993). Interrater agreement of visual analysis in single-subject, decisions: Quantitative review and analysis. *American Journal of Mental Retardation, 98*, 135–142.

Pedley, K., Giles, E., & Hogan, A. (2005). *Adult cochlear implant rehabilitation*. Philadelphia: Whurr.

Pratt, S. R., Heintzelman, A. T., & Deming, S. E. (1993). The efficacy of using the IBM speech viewer vowel accuracy module to treat young children with hearing impairment. *Journal of Speech and Hearing Research, 36*, 1063–1074.

Proops, D. W. (2006) The cochlear implant team. In H. R. Cooper & L. C. Craddock (Eds.), *Cochlear implants: A practical guide* (2nd ed., pp. 70–79). West Sussex: Whurr.

Rebmann, M. J., & Hannon, R. (1995). Treatment of unawareness of memory deficits in adults with brain injury: Three case studies. *Rehabilitation Psychology, 40*(4), 279–287.

Robey, R. R., Schultz, M. C., Crawford, A. B., & Sinner, C. A. (1999). Single-subject clinical-outcome research: Designs, data, effect sizes, and analyses. *Aphasiology, 13*, 445–473.

Satake, E. (1994). Bayesian inference in polling technique: 1992 Presidential polls, *Communication Research, 21*(3), 396–407.

Simpson, M. B., Till, J. A., & Goff, A. M. (1988). Long-term treatment of severe dysarthria: A case study. *Journal of Speech and Hearing Disorders, 53*, 433–440.

Tawney, J. W., & Gast, D. L. (1984). *Single subject research in special education*. Columbus, OH: Charles Merrill.

Todman, J. B., & Dugard, P. (2001). *Single-case and small-n experimental design: A practical guide to randomization tests*. Mahwah, NJ: Erlbaum.

Tomblin, J. B., Spencer, L., Flock, S., Tyler, R., & Gantz, B. (1999). A comparison of language achievement in children with cochlear implants and children using hearing aids. *Journal of Speech, Language, and Hearing Research, 42*(2), 497–509.

Tye-Murray, N., Spencer, L., Bedia, E. G., & Woodworth, G. (1996). Differences in children's sound production when speaking with a cochlear implant turned on and turned off. *Journal of Speech and Hearing Research, 39*(3), 604–610.

Tyler, R. S., Fryauf-Bertschy, H., Kelsay, D. M., Gantz, B. J., Woodworth, G. P., & Parkinson, A. (1997). Speech perception by prelingually deaf children using cochlear implants. *Otolaryngology-Head And Neck Surgery, 117*(3, Pt. 1), 180–187.

Waltzman, S. B., & Cohen, N. L. (2000). *Cochlear implants*. New York: Thieme Medical.

Wambaugh, J., Cameron, R., Kalinyak-Fliszar, M., Nessler, C., & Wright, S. (2004). Retrieval of action names in aphasia: Effects of two cueing treatments. *Aphasiology, 18*(11), 979–1004.

Watling, R., Deitz, J., Kanny, E. M., & McLaughlin, J. F. (1999). Current practice of occupational therapy for children with autism. *American Journal of Occupational Therapy, 53*(5), 498–505.

Wimpory, D., Chadwick, P., & Nash, S. (1995). Brief report: Musical interaction therapy for children with autism: An evaluative case study with two-year follow-up. *Journal of Autism and Developmental Disorders, 25*(5), 541–552.

Yorkston, K. M. (1996). Treatment efficacy: Dysarthria. *Journal of Speech and Hearing Research, 39*(5), S46–S57.

Yorkston, K. M., Beukelman, D. R., & Bell, K. R. (1988). *Clinical management of dysarthric speakers*. Austin, TX: Pro-Ed.

Young, M. C. (2003). Anterior aphasia as a natural category of acquired cognitive-communicative impairment: Implications for cognitive neurolinguistic theory, experimental methods, and clinical practice. *Dissertation Abstracts International, 64*(5-B), 2415.

Index